HOLISTIC SKINCARE

AN ESSENTIAL GUIDE FOR THERAPISTS

ANGELA EGAN

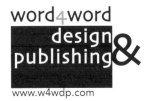

www.w4wdp.com

Acknowledgements

I would like to thank my Mother and my long-suffering sisters, Elizabeth and Margaret, who allowed me to bully them about their skincare, and who tolerated hours of experimental 'treatments' in the pursuit of healthy, glowing skin.

To Angi Hall, for her unbelievable patience during my holistic therapy training but mostly for her discipline, passion and commitment to the standards and knowledge needed to become an outstanding therapist - her example has been a constant inspiration and benchmark for all I endeavour to achieve.

To the countless therapists I have had the pleasure of teaching and learning from - this book is a testimony to your thirst for knowledge and an acknowledgement of the amazing talents you all have. You're working in the most diverse and wonderful industry in the world; congratulations for having the wisdom to become involved!

My gorgeous partner, Graham, who suggested I should write a book in the first place, who encourages me with kind words (and technical support when gremlins sneak into my laptop!) and who offers constant support and enduring love. Thank you for teaching me the principles of perseverance and rock-solid self-belief. Most of all for being wise enough to retain a child-like heart - great is the man.

Finally to Sue Richardson at Word4Word Design & Publishing Ltd whose knowledge and experience in design and publishing have made this part of the journey truly five star. The greatest joy was discovering a publisher who intuitively and effortlessly understood the vision I had for the book, and what I wanted it to communicate. Best of all has been working with an accomplished master of their profession - it makes life bliss!

To Monty and Maisy - whom I love with all my heart.

ABOUT THE AUTHOR

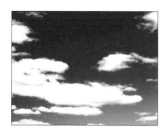

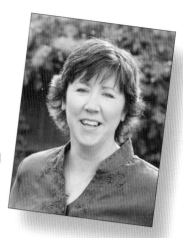

Angela has had a fascination for skincare since late childhood when she intuitively used ingredients from the family kitchen to pamper her sisters and herself with naturally created face and hair packs. As the youngest of six children, Angela did not have money to waste, but instead had to rely upon the family's own natural resources and the harvest from the garden, which provided a wealth of fruits, vegetables and herbs. She had an insatiable curiosity for discovering the effect particular ingredients had on the skin and was famed for 'messing about in the bathroom' rather than watching TV.

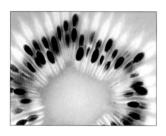

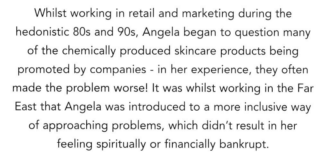

Whilst working in retail and marketing during the hedonistic 80s and 90s, Angela began to question many of the chemically produced skincare products being promoted by companies - in her experience, they often made the problem worse! It was whilst working in the Far East that Angela was introduced to a more inclusive way of approaching problems, which didn't result in her feeling spiritually or financially bankrupt.

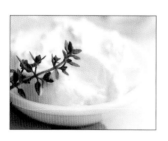

This started a fascination and commitment to study holistic medicine and in 1999 Angela qualified as a Holistic Practitioner working with a diverse range of people in private health clubs, spas and natural health practices. She continues to teach skincare specialists, holistic therapists and clients on the benefits of becoming a 'label detective' in the field of skincare and nutrition.

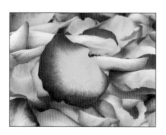

Finally, Angela has a wonderful way of empowering people to take responsibility for their own well-being.

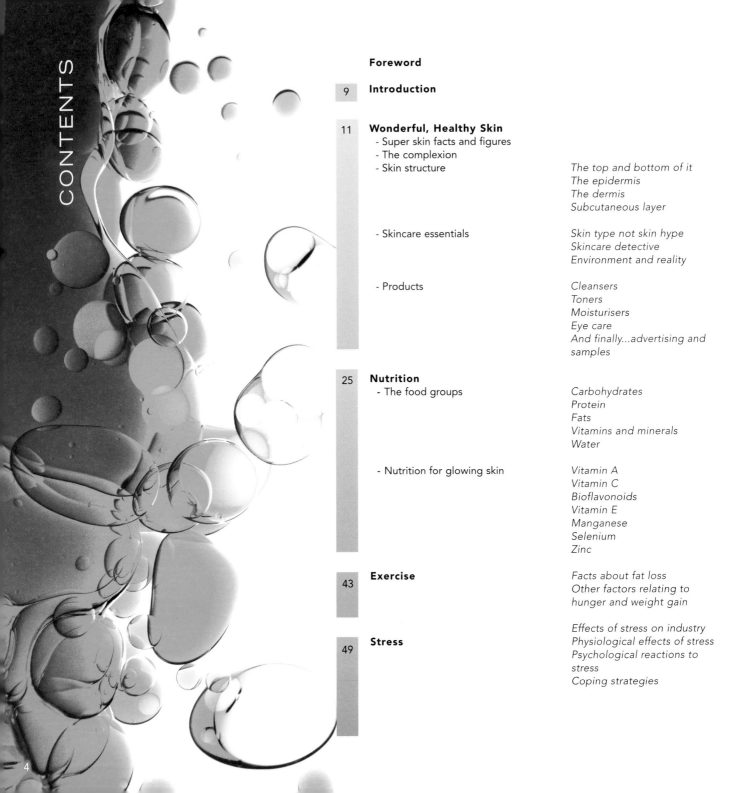

CONTENTS

"It's not who we are that holds us back, it's who we think we're not"

Michael Nolan

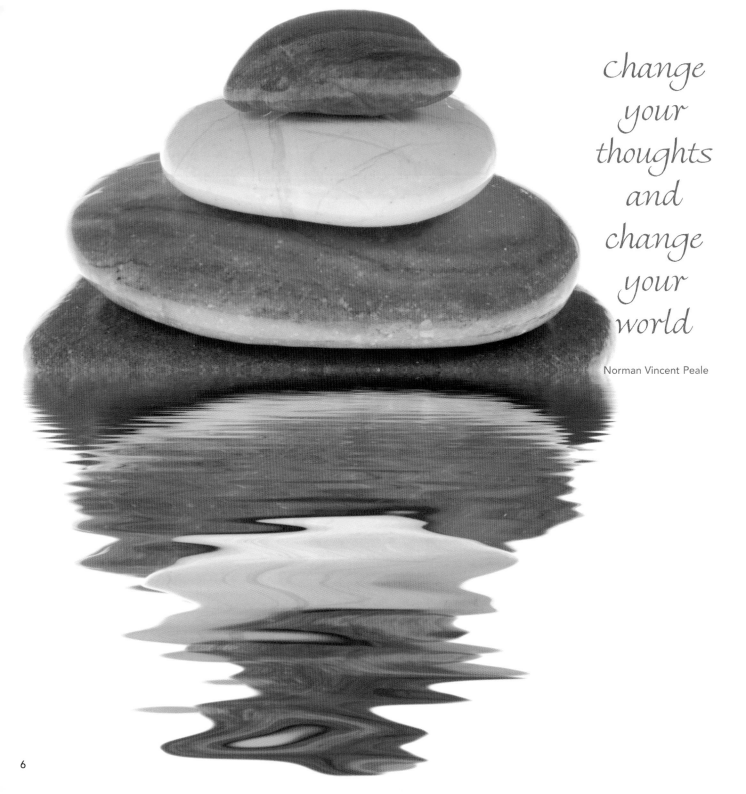

change
your
thoughts
and
change
your
world

Norman Vincent Peale

FOREWORD

When I became a beauty therapist some 27 years ago it was very clear to me from the onset that beauty was so much more than just skin deep. It made perfect sense to me that beauty, health and well-being were intrinsically linked.

How could anyone expect to look or feel beautiful if they did not feel it from within? It was on that basis I decided to incorporate holistic therapies into my traditional beauty therapies; I knew this way it would be easier to get the desired effect I knew I could achieve as a therapist.

I drew from my Indian heritage and upbringing and began to incorporate no-nonsense Ayurvedic principles into my business. This meant not only in the treatments but also in the form of sound advice that a person could take away with them and use in their day-to-day lives.

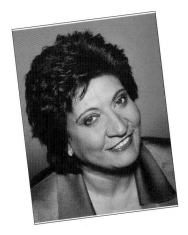

Bharti Vyas
Holistic Beauty Therapist

Passing knowledge onto the client is a fantastic way to help boost society's health and well-being too. This makes our roles as holistic therapists so much more valuable and satisfying. I think it's a really exciting time to be in the health and beauty industry; whilst we are continually advancing our knowledge we are able to positively enhance the lives of our clients. Gone are the days when therapists were seen as brainless – we are now so much more than that and I for one am very proud to be in the industry.

On top of this, there is vast array of knowledge available to us. Angela's book provides an excellent guide for therapists, whilst being beautifully illustrated and highly informative. More so, it allows those of us working in the profession to consider which disciplines support our practice and which we feel will be of most value to our clients. I can see holistic therapies continuing to play a pivotal role in the beauty industry. Books like this make it so much easier for us all.

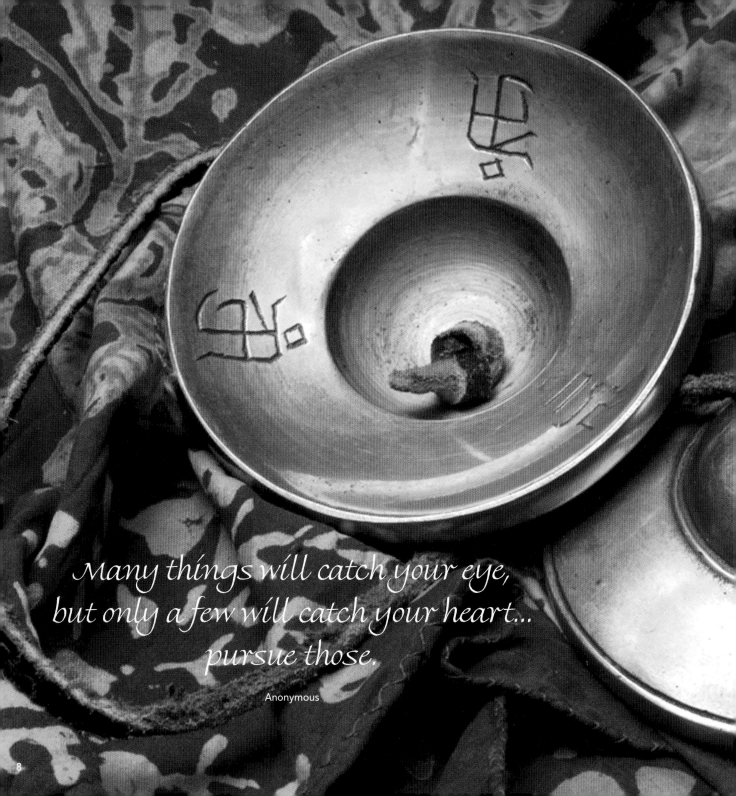

Many things will catch your eye,
but only a few will catch your heart...
pursue those.

Anonymous

INTRODUCTION

As the demands of being a holistic skincare specialist increase so does the client's knowledge and expectations of immediate results. At a time when high-technology cosmeceuticals are making procedures such as botox, chemical peels and dermabrasion increasingly mainstream, the client wants more than just traditional skincare.

However, although the barriers are being pushed further back, it seems paradoxical that holistic medicine is also enjoying an extraordinary renaissance.

This is the first edition of a comprehensive holistic skincare therapist handbook, which can be read from cover to cover or can be dipped into whenever the need occurs.

Either way, enjoy the aims of this book.

I hope to de-mystify the complexities and ambiguities of holistic medicine, and to encourage you to ask questions of yourselves and your clients that will lead to the safest, most effective and beneficial treatment for them.

You can also register for my quarterly newsletter by visiting www.purevisionuk.com where you are welcome to contribute ideas, comments and experiences, ask questions and debate the evolving world of the holistic skincare therapist.

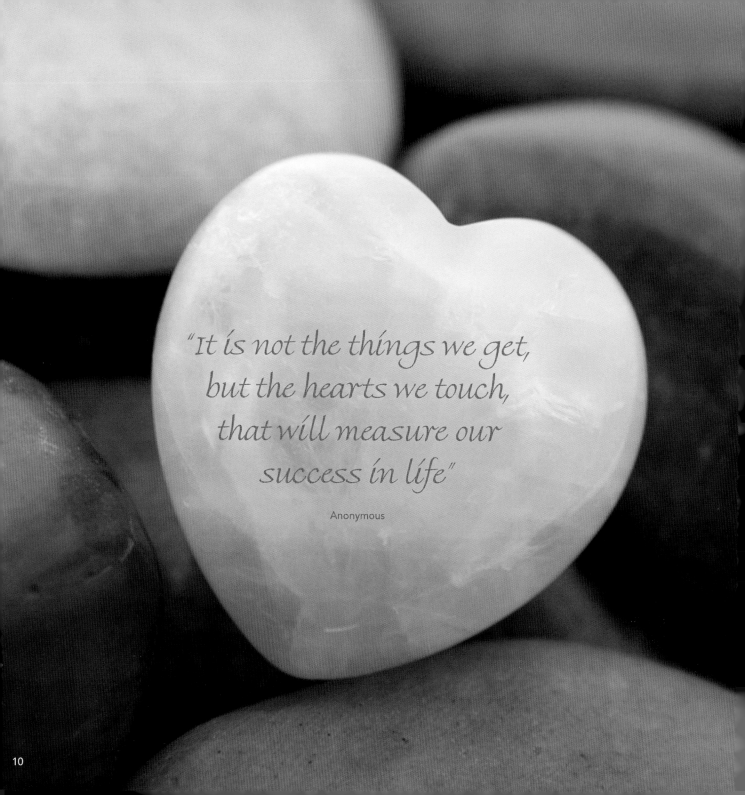

"It is not the things we get,
but the hearts we touch,
that will measure our
success in life"

Anonymous

WONDERFUL, HEALTHY SKIN

Super Skin Facts and Figures

The skin is more than a convenient layer separating you from the outside world. The skin is our largest organ, with a range of functions that support our survival. Let's remind ourselves how amazing the skin's structure is. As the body's largest organ, if spread out it would cover about 2 square meters, it is approximately 0.5mm thick around the eyes to 6mm thick or more on the soles of the feet, and weighs anything from 2.75 to 4 kilograms.

This wonderful organ is waterproof, washable and 'like wax paper, it holds everything in without dripping'. Art Linkletter

It acts as a temperature regulator, a major route for the elimination of toxins, produces vitamin D and, given the right nutrients, has the incredible capacity to heal itself and act as an efficient defender against trauma, infection and invasion.

Finally, if the eyes are the windows to our soul, the skin is definitely the barometer of our inner health.

The Complexion

When we look at our reflections in the mirror, the first thing we usually see is the condition of our skin.

Our general complexion - commonly judged by the skin on our face and cheeks - is the most visual indicator of our overall health. When the mind and body are in a state of balance, or homeostasis, we have a natural capacity for self-regulation and repair.

The ability to maintain this equilibrium can be overwhelmed when placed under strain, either emotionally or physically, resulting in greater demands being placed upon the 'whole' and so affecting the balance of the other parts. For example, long-term emotional tension can result in chronic physical fatigue. A stressful lifestyle, lack of sleep and a diet low in the essential vitamins and minerals will eventually show in a person's complexion.

It is therefore essential to address the 'whole person' when looking at the skin and using this knowledge to advise your clients authoritatively. In my experience, a person's greatest loyalty has been realised when they have received both an understanding and an empathy of their 'unspoken self' simply by interpreting their skin.

Once you study the skin in detail, you'll begin to see how magnificent but highly complicated it is.

Skin Structure

~ The top and bottom of it ~

Holding in mind the importance of the skin, it is worth reminding ourselves that the body's largest organ is not an unstructured bundle of cells but a complicated structure. The skin consists of two layers: the epidermis on the outside and the dermis on the inside.

The main function of the epidermis is to offer protection against the outside elements through a tough barrier, whilst the dermis is a thick, soft cushion of connective tissue that lies directly beneath the epidermis. It determines how the skin looks and is the active part of the skin, holding the hair muscles, blood supply, subcutaneous glands and nerve receptors.

Both layers are constantly renewing and repairing themselves, with the dermis doing so more slowly than the epidermis. This is because skin cells are reproducing all the time, with new cells being created in the lower dermis by cell division. They then move towards the surface where they eventually die and flake off.

This process takes about 28 days to complete but slows down with ageing, although cellular renewal can be stimulated by certain plant extracts and essential oils (see Aromatherapy chapter). Think of the wonderful luminance present in a child's skin (that is frankly wasted on the young) and which is desired and highly prized in adulthood!

Below the dermis is a layer of fat cells, known as adipose tissue, or subcutaneous fat, which provides a source of energy, insulation and a protective cushion.

~ The epidermis ~

In the epidermis, the cells become flatter and are keratinised, which makes them tougher and waterproof. The top layer of the skin is the stratum corneum (horny layer). It is the layer of the skin we see from the outside and, being distant from the blood supply in the dermis, is principally made up of dead, flaky skin.

These dead skin cells are continually shed from the skin's surface, and this is balanced by the production of new ones in the stratum germinativium (basal) layer. Also in the basal layer are melanocyte cells that produce melanin, our protection against ultraviolet light.

~ The dermis ~

Below the epidermis is the layer called the dermis. The top layer of the dermis - the one directly below the epidermis - has many ridges called papillae. On the fingertips, the skin's surface follows this pattern of ridges to create our individual fingerprints.

The dermis contains a variable amount of fat and also collagen and elastin fibres, which give strength and flexibility to the skin. In an older person, the elastin fibres fragment and much of the skin's elasticity is lost. This results in creases and wrinkles becoming a permanent feature in the skin.

Collagen and elastin are the skin's natural scaffolding, with collagen accounting for 75% of the skin's structure and elastin around 5%. Together they are responsible for the skin's structure and shape, its smoothness, strength and elasticity. So it's pretty apparent that collagen and elastin are responsible for the health and appearance of our skin. Another amazing capability of collagen and elastin is that they can easily regenerate, which is why the skin can repair and heal so quickly.

sweat pore — hair
epidermis
dermis
sebaceous glands
sweat gland
subcutaneous layer
venous blood
arterial blood

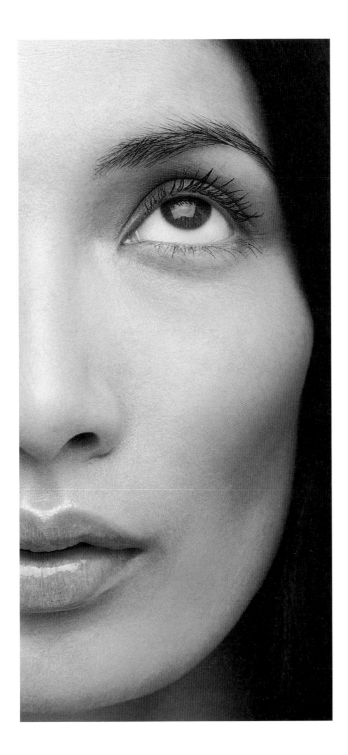

Blood vessels also supply nutrients to the dividing cells in the basal layer and remove any waste products. These blood vessels also help to maintain the body's temperature by dilating and carrying more blood when the body needs to lose heat from its surface.

Specialised nerves in the dermis detect heat, cold, pain, touch and pressure and relay this information to the brain - this way the body senses changes in the environment that may potentially cause harm.

Hair follicles are embedded in the dermis and occur all over the body except in the soles of the feet, palms of the hand and lips. Attached to each hair follicle are small erector pili muscle fibres, which contract in cold weather and fright; this pulls the hair up, which pulls on the skin resulting in goose bumps being visible.

A sebaceous (oil) gland opens into each hair follicle and produces sebum, a lubricant for the hair and skin that helps repel water, damaging chemicals and micro-organisms, or germs. This is also responsible for maintaining the skin's first defence - the acid mantle - this has a pH balance of between 5 and 6 and is easily disrupted by harsh skincare products such as those containing SD alcohols and acetone derivatives.

Sweat glands occur on all areas of the skin, in fact each of us has more than 2 million, and, when the body needs to lose heat, these glands produce sweat - this moves to the surface of the skin via the sweat duct, and the evaporation of this water from the skin has a cooling effect on the body. These sweat glands are also responsible for assisting with the removal of waste material such as urea and so play a part in the body's elimination process.

There are two types of sweat gland - eccrine and appocrine - the eccrine occur all over the body, with more on the hands and feet, and produce a watery substance (sweat). Appocrine glands are present only in the axillae (arm pits) and the groin; they produce a milky substance and are responsible for our 'natural' body odour, known as ferazomes.

~ Subcutaneous layer (adipose tissue) ~

The innermost cover of the skin is the layer of subcutaneous fat or adipose tissue, and its thickness varies in regions of the body. Evolution has also deemed that females have more adipose tissue than men, particularly around the hips and buttocks – sorry about that, ladies. The stored fat represents an energy source for the body and helps to insulate against changes in the outside temperature as well as acting as protection for vital organs.

Skincare Essentials

~ Skin type not skin hype ~

One of the most distorted skincare concepts present in the industry today is the notion of a permanent skin type. The way we are educated as therapists about skin type categories is often too rigid, and this is further reinforced by an industry persuading us to buy these products. All too often asking a client about their skin type informs the advice we offer them and this advice may not be the most helpful – for their skin or your reputation.

The principal difficulty in determining a clients' skin type is that in addition to their general skin condition, many outside factors can, and do, influence what their skin feels like and how things appear on the day they come to you for a treatment.

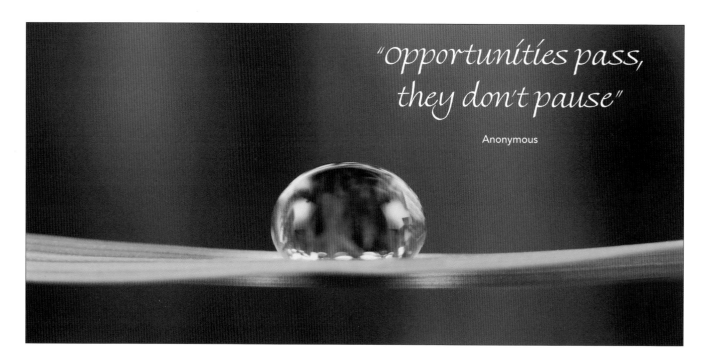

"opportunities pass, they don't pause"

Anonymous

It is a fairly pointless exercise trying to rationally discuss skincare needs until you have established what other causes exist that may be affecting their skin health. Consideration needs to be given to factors such as using irritating and harsh skincare products, poor nutrition, lack of exercise, unmanaged stress, smoking, excess alcohol, exposing skin to sun with no protection (or other forms of UVA light), free-radical damage... and so the list goes on.

A final point on skin-types is the modern day phenomena of sensitive skin. Everyone has sensitive skin at some time or another. The role of a professional skincare therapist is to discover what has caused the skin to become sensitised in the first place, and stop the client using it! Countless times I have asked clients with sensitive skin what they are using and how long they have been using it. If they have been using a product marketed specifically for sensitive skin for a number of years I will innocently ask why their skin remains sensitive?

In other words, they need to be treating or combating the issue, and it's the role of the skincare therapist to suggest products that can do just that.

More often than not two ingredients commonly added to skincare products are often thought to be the main causes – fragrance and preservatives. These can cause the skin to burn, tingle, flake, itch, breakout into bumps & pimples, or become red or sore.

Preservatives are impossible to avoid, and mandatory under European legislation – without them products become mouldy and full of bacteria. However there are numerous naturally occurring preservatives that are far less irritating on the skin.

Fragrance smells nice but has absolutely no place in effective facial skincare so should be avoided at all costs.

The instruction for sensitive skin is the same for oily, acne prone, dry or maturing – treat the skin as gently as possible and avoid things that cause irritation. Try recommending they use fewer products with smaller ingredient lists and I believe the sensitivity issue will cease to exist.

~ *Skincare detective* ~

To concentrate exclusively on skin type is at best misleading, and at worst highly damaging to your reputation as a skincare specialist. Concentrating on this makes the skincare advice you offer obsolete, even before the client has arrived home.

It is possible, and not at all unusual, to have simultaneously different skin types during any given week or month. As a therapist you must take into consideration not only a clients physical environment but also factors such as the current climate, their lifestyle, menstrual cycle, weight fluctuations, their stress levels (this affects the hormones, which in turn affects the skin), their 'emotional' health and then the condition of the skin as you see and feel it.

Becoming a skincare detective requires detailed and thorough investigations but it means the advice you offer is then based on a sound and holistic understanding of their individual needs and requirements. And your client is always worth it.

~ *Environment and reality* ~

The kind of environment a client lives and works in most definitely has an effect on the skin. Those living and working in polluted cities and air-conditioned environments will most certainly

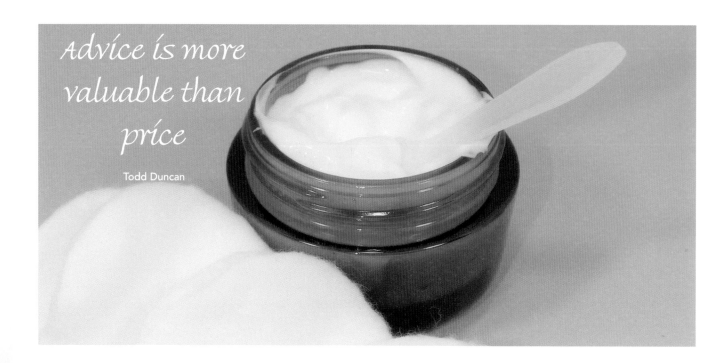

Advice is more valuable than price

Todd Duncan

present with different skincare needs to someone who lives in open countryside or by the sea.

Their current skincare routine will also play a significant part in the current condition of the skin. Too many unsuitable skincare products will create confusion and distort the facts. An overuse of AHAs, BHAs, excessive use of overly-abrasive exfoliators and incorrect moisturisers all adversely affect the skin.

Your role is to gently describe how the current use of soap to wash with, alcohol-based wipes, perfumed cleanser, perfume based moisturiser, or whatever it is that is responsible for their existing skin condition needs to be replaced with something you can recommend. More of how to do this without offending later.

Products

~ Cleansers ~

Water-soluble and nothing else
The best advice to offer a client regarding the cleansing routine is that they chose one to fit in with their current lifestyle. As soon as you get into the realms of clients having to alter their existing skincare routine, especially allocating more time, you are setting them up for disillusionment and a return to their potentially damaging skincare habits.

Secondly, the cleanser must be gentle and water-soluble – this is true for all skin types. If the client does not use a water-soluble cleanser to remove make-up, impurities and daily grime, then the residue that remains from the cleanser can clog pores and prevent skin-cells from sloughing off.

Using a cleanser that leaves a greasy film on the face can not only clog pores but also prevent moisturisers from being absorbed and doing their job.

It is essential to get this step right, and that means thoroughly, yet gently, cleansing the skin.

~ Toners ~

Tea-total skincare

Toners are described and marketed under several different names by skincare companies, for example, astringents, clarifiers, refiners, fresheners and tonics. In reality, toners don't tone anything but can help to prepare the skin for a moisturiser or serum.

Toners of any kind will not firm the skin, they won't deep clean, and they won't close pores. What well-formulated toners can do however is reduce inflammation, add moisturising factors to the skin, and help remove the last traces of make-up residue.

Advise clients to avoid all toners containing SD alcohol and acetone (nail varnish remover for goodness sake!), fragrance, any citrus oils, camphor, mint, menthol, and high levels of witch hazel – all of these ingredients can make the skin sensitive, leading to irritation and should therefore be avoided.

~ Moisturisers ~

A challenge to your thinking

All cosmetic skincare companies would have you believe that the health of our skin is dependant upon a moisturiser, and most skincare therapists have been taught this in a mantra-like fashion. It simply isn't true. Not everyone needs a moisturiser, especially those with combination and acne-prone skin. Moisturiser, and the selling of it, is one of the most misused and abused areas of skincare.

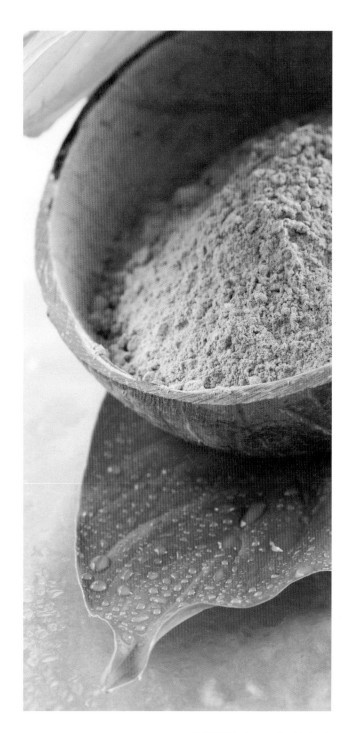

Moisturisers are often way overpriced, have massively exaggerated claims attached to them, and are often responsible for the skin concern your client presents with!

Where the skin has dry patches, apply a moisturiser. Clients don't need to use it all over, unless the skin is dry all over - and chances are this is being caused by something else they're using. If clients don't have dry skin, don't recommend they use a moisturiser. It's that simple. Encourage them to monitor their skin: it may be that their skin is fine during the summer but needs extra moisture in the winter.

The dreaded wrinkles

Using a moisturiser is fine for smoothing out the appearance of lines and wrinkles (they won't change the wrinkle, they'll just smooth it out) but using a moisturiser will not prevent wrinkles. A moisturiser, irrespective of the cost or ingredients, will not firm, tone, repair or lift the skin despite what claims are made. Many clients, and alarmingly some therapists, still support the mistaken belief that moisturisers somehow prevent wrinkles. More alarmingly is the belief that failing to use a moisturiser will somehow give you wrinkles, or that dry skin is naturally more prone to wrinkled skin than oily skin - both are without foundation.

Those moisturisers with an SPF such as titanium dioxide, zinc oxide et al will limit further skin damage but won't reverse wrinkles caused by sun damage.

Recognising that a client doesn't need a moisturiser doesn't mean their skin won't benefit from products containing a sunscreen, an anti-irritant, antioxidant or other emollient, water-binding, humectant-type product.

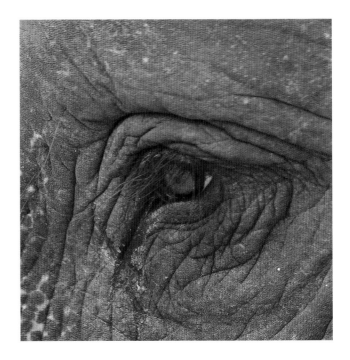

If you have recommended they use a gentle cleanser with great moisturising ingredients (essential fatty acids, and jojoba, olive, almond, avocado and wheat germ oil to name a few) followed by a toner that doesn't strip the skin by using SD alcohol or acetone, then a moisturiser may not be necessary; many foundations also contain effective moisturisers so that clients can easily hydrate their skin without layers of unnecessary products.

~ Eye care ~

Less is definitely more where the skin around the eye area is concerned as this is where the skin is thinnest and most delicate. It has no sebaceous glands and is one of the first areas of the face to show signs of stress and ageing through wrinkles, dark shadows under the eyes and puffiness.

A number of factors can also cause eye strain, including excessive driving, reading, working with VDU screens and watching TV. Air pollution and fatigue can also cause or aggravate eye strain.

When a client's eyes are strained or aching, it is often a signal that they are under stress and the whole body is fatigued. They will probably also be irritable, suffer from headaches and be tight across the neck and shoulders. When performing a facial or back, neck and shoulder massage, it is probably a good idea to spend extra time applying pressure to the points associated with eye strain and tension. This is generally met with a cry of approval from your client who explains it is painful, but in a strangely nice way! (See diagrams 1 and 2 for pressure points.)

One of the traditions in Ayurvedic medicine is the bathing of the eye itself, around the eye and even the focusing on beautiful things to relieve the eye. Practitioners advocate bathing the eyes in cool water or rose water every morning to keep them healthy, although this is to be done with the eyes open. This is followed once a week with an eyebath or eyecup containing 3-5 drops of ghee

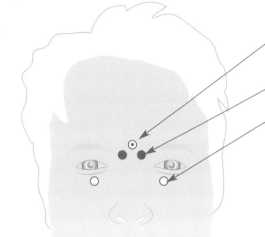

> This helps with the endocrine system - also hayfever, headaches and eyestrain.
> Relieves red, painful eyes, headaches, eyestrain.
> Relieves burning or aching eyes, foggy vision & hayfever.

Diagram 1

> At the top of the spinal column in the large hollow of the skull. Great for relieving tension headaches.
> Either side of the cervical spine. Relieves stress, burn-out, exhaustion, swollen eyes and eyestrain.

Diagram 2

(clarified butter). Following the eyebath, the ghee would then be gently massaged into the skin under and around the eyes, ending the ritual with some pinching along the eyebrows and gentle pressures on the eye socket - always moving from the inside to the outside.

Eye cleansing

Gentle but meticulous cleansing is required with purpose-made products, which should be water-soluble and free from fragrance, artificial colouring and SD alcohol. Where a client has concerns over their eye area, I have generally found they are using 'just my normal cleanser', they are using products that are too harsh, or they are too heavy-handed when removing eye make-up. Worse still is the client who doesn't bother to remove their make-up each night. It is worth explaining that this causes inflammation and irritation, which leads to swelling and a puffy appearance around the eyes.

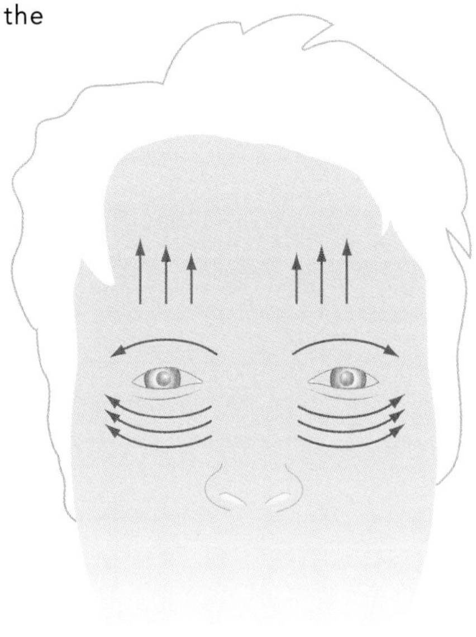

Any time a client is rubbing, pulling and stretching the delicate skin around the eye area, they are weakening muscle structure along with damaging elastin and collagen fibres; all guaranteed to accelerate the signs of ageing.

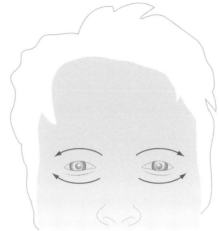

> Apply a light pressure using 'pads' of fingers.
> Only apply to boney eye socket area avoiding the eyelid and directly beneath the eye

Diagram 3

> Sliding drain movements to begin.
> Followed by pumping movements.
> Pressure to be gentle and featherlike.

Diagram 4

Eye creams

Whether your client is using an eye gel or eye cream, they will generally be using too much product. Most will have had visible results with the small amount recommended by you initially, and so will be tempted to use more in the belief that this will generate even better results. We all know this is wrong, but I figure we've all done it - I certainly have!

Most clients have a plethora of failed eye products. My experience is that on almost every occasion the application, not the product, has been the problem. The best investment you'll make with a client will be taking time to explain how and where to apply an eye product.

Care must be taken to use the ring finger for application (it's harder to apply a heavy pressure using this finger compared to your index finger) and then only ever apply to the eye socket area. (See diagram 3.)

Most clients will introduce product to the eyelid and directly under the eye. This can set up a histamine reaction due to the product seeping into the tear duct and down the hair follicle of the eyelashes - hence the client waking up the following morning looking like the bog-eyed monster they were trying to banish!

Bags and dark circles

Bags under the eyes are usually inherited but regular physical exercise can help to reduce them. Exercise helps to carry oxygen to the skin cells and removes waste. If you can encourage clients to make time in the morning to apply a cool compress on the eyes (low temperatures make the skin contract), this will help. If time really doesn't allow, suggest the client keeps their eye cream or moisturiser in the fridge so it is cool when applied in the morning.

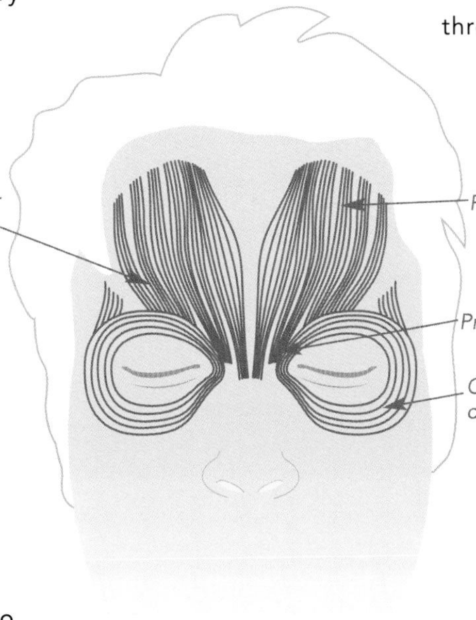

In traditional Chinese medicine, the area under the eye relates to the liver, an organ responsible for (amongst many other things) the filtering of toxins and the detoxifying of drugs. When, through the stresses of general lifestyle choices, poor nutrition, or a course of medication, the liver becomes overwhelmed and starts to operate a little sluggishly (rather like not cleaning the filter on an air-conditioning unit), extra help is needed.

Advising your client about foods that act as great liver and kidney cleansers and also explaining the benefits of light massage and gentle acupressure each day, can go a long way to help relieve bags under the eyes and dark circles. Take time to demonstrate to them the benefits of some manual lymphatic drainage (MLD) movements and you will have a client for life. (See diagram 4).

The bigger picture

Lastly, clients will naturally concentrate their efforts and energy directly onto the eye area, because this is what they're concerned about. Your role is to remind them of the connecting parts that help lift or harm the muscle structure. Remembering that

Corrugator

Frontalis

Procerus

Orbicularis oculi

Diagram 5

muscles pull rather than push, and that all muscles work in antagonistic pairs, it is helpful to physically demonstrate to a client what you mean. Try raising your eyebrows in surprise and see what effect this has on the surrounding eye area. In the same way, try frowning and see how many wrinkles this creates!

Gentle massage and manual lifting of the large frontalis muscle helps relieve tension in the face and smoothes out fine lines across the forehead. Incorporate the corrugator and procerus muscles to help relieve lines caused by continual frowning. Finally, massage the orbicularis oculi muscle to smooth out crow's feet, the principal causes of which being squinting and frowning. (See diagram 5.)

~ And finally... advertising and samples ~

We all know that advertisers pay huge sums of money to sell more products - nothing wrong with that, some might say. Where it becomes more difficult is where the advertisers use misleading messages to seduce consumers by playing on our vulnerabilities and insecurities.

I am endlessly fascinated by the advertising small print for skincare products, which often state in the tiniest print that the 'scientific tests' were 'carried out on 30 women', using 'self-evaluation', or compared to 'unmoisturised skin'. This is the equivalent of tests with vodka to see if it gets people drunk, those who drank it got drunk, those who didn't drink it remained sober - no surprises there then!

One of the reasons clients are seduced by misleading advertising claims is the endless media formats they use to communicate their message. Very quickly this repetitive, consistent message

gives credibility, authority and confidence to the customer - I know, I've been using the same principle for years as a Visual Merchandiser! It also suggests that we are missing out on something if we haven't tried the product yet.

As a skincare specialist, you need to be aware of this when you are helping your client understand that the product being advertised is the very one that is responsible for the concern they have. You need to be just as authoritative and confident in your communication.

Samples are an area where skincare specialists unwittingly undermine their own credibility. Having spent time with a client, either during a great facial or on a one-to-one in the retail area, we are in the best position ever to deliver authoritative advice based on the facts from what the client has said, and also from what we can see.

So we have listened to the problem and, as the qualified, knowledgeable therapist, we have matched this with the best solution. We then offer a sample rather than a product. It is the equivalent of confidently saying 'I would recommend X product because I know it will help this problem' and then ending with 'However, I might be wrong, so try a sample first'.

Please don't misunderstand me - I believe samples are a wonderful way of introducing link products to a purchasing client, just not as a 'try before you buy' method of retailing. Use them for marketing, not for undermining your credibility.

Another reason I feel so strongly about the use of samples by professional therapists is the fact that the skin renews itself over a 28-day cycle. Therefore, it stands to reason that we need to use a

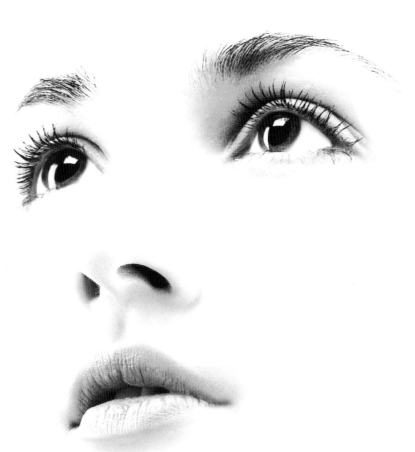

product for this amount of time before we can be absolutely sure it is the right one (excepting immediate allergic reactions, of course). Most samples only ever last five to six days, and sometimes just one application. I know from experience that I have made expensive mistakes by purchasing products after using the sample, only to discover in a month or two that the product isn't right for me.

Healthy skin and beauty go hand in hand, and the skin reflects our health and inner feelings. The best way to achieve optimum skin health is by taking time out every day for ourselves. Skin is like a mirror - it reflects everything that's happening inside the body and the mind. When we've had enough rest, then high energy levels and general well-being will be reflected in glowing skin and clear bright eyes.

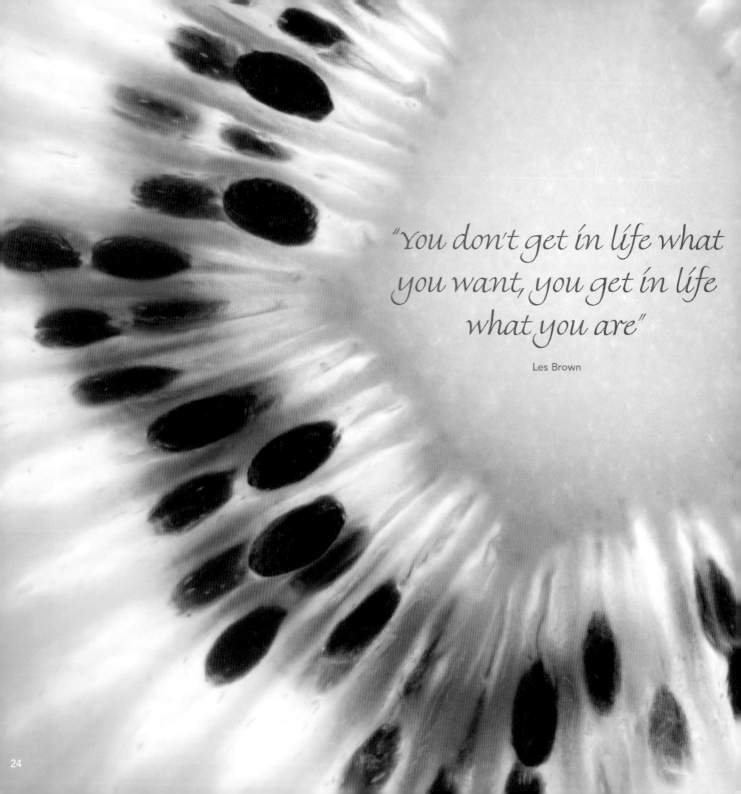

"You don't get in life what you want, you get in life what you are"

Les Brown

NUTRITION

What we eat and what we drink really are vital parts of what we are - and what we will become. Along with rest and relaxation, a nutritious diet is one of the essential ways we can protect and nourish our skin. Everything we do (and don't) put into our mouths is likely to affect optimum skin health.

The amazing thing is that many of the skin problems your client presents with can be completely transformed by making straightforward but hugely beneficial changes to the diet. Greater emphasis needs to be placed on treating skin problems from the inside (from nutrition) than by the use of creams and lotions from the outside.

For example

- A clogged, spotty complexion often reveals a diet high in unhealthy fats and sugar

- An ultra-sensitive skin may be the result of poor digestion and inadequate absorption of nutrients

- Very dry, flaky skin may indicate deficiencies of essential fatty acids (EFAs) and vitamin E

- Slow-healing skin may need vitamins A and B6, and zinc

In this chapter, we shall look at skin helpers and skin villains, nutritional supplements, basic food groups and eating the right food combinations.

For the benefit of skin health we need to make full use of Mother Nature's healing sustenance, including fresh fruit and vegetables, nuts, seeds, wholegrains, fresh fish - and masses of fresh water!

The skin foods detailed here are a selection of some of the best.

The Food Groups

Nutritional experts all advocate a balanced diet that includes a wide variety from the main food groups every day.

1. Carbohydrates
2. Protein
3. Fats
4. Vitamins
5. Minerals
6. Fibre
7. Liquids such as water and juices

Eating a variety of foods from each of the groups should satisfy most nutritional requirements. The key to a balanced diet is the correct amount of proteins, carbohydrates and fats. Vegetables should make up the dominant part of any diet, with fish and fruit being the other vital components.

~ Carbohydrates ~

What do they do?
Carbohydrates are the body's primary source of energy and the main fuel for the body's cellular renewal. They're used in the brain, nervous system and muscles. Carbohydrates, which include sugars, starches and cellulose, also help to break down and burn fat.

These are the plant foods that not only supply your body with an easily converted form of energy but also contain other vital nutrients. They have few health drawbacks, and 'spare' protein from having to be converted into energy (protein is needed for growth, repair and maintenance of the body - this is its primary role).

Once broken down by the digestive system, carbohydrates are stored in the liver and the muscles as glycogen. The liver can store about a fist full of carbohydrates from any one meal. Any more than this will be stored as fat.

What are they?

Carbohydrates can be digestible or indigestible; the indigestible part is called fibre. Complex carbohydrates provide fibre, as well as sugar and starch, which is important because it helps to slow the release of sugars into the blood stream, which stabilises blood sugar levels. The digestible part is broken down by the body into energy-giving sugar. This enables us to remain alert and energised throughout the day.

Fibre is also needed for regular bowel movements. It acts as the body's vacuum cleaner, clearing out toxins that may have crept into our bodies from foods or smoking. A daily intake of 30 grams of fibre is recommended.

What's the best source of carbohydrate?

The best sources of complex carbohydrates feature fruits, vegetables, brown rice, wholegrain pasta, wholegrain bread, potatoes, rye crackers, oat and buckwheat noodles.

Avoid simple carbohydrates, often referred to as fast release. These include sweets, chocolates, sugary drinks, white rice, white pasta and white bread. They contain very little indigestible fibre and so are broken down quickly, releasing a rush of sugar into the blood stream. After an initial rush of energy, you may experience a low that makes you feel even worse than you did before you ate. This is because the rush results in low energy and blood sugar levels. In an attempt to stabilise blood sugar levels your body craves more of these foods and the cycle continues.

How much do I need?

Complex carbohydrates should make up 55% of your daily nutritional intake. Eating an evening meal low in starchy carbohydrates, such as potatoes and bread, but high in carbohydrates from vegetable and fruit sources, can help with fat loss.

For weight management, it is recommended that roughly a third of your main meal consists of complex carbohydrates, such as easy cooked brown rice, red rice, buckwheat noodles, wholegrain pasta or potato; a third comprises vegetables or salad; and a third should contain meat, fish, soya or tofu.

Digestible carbohydrates may be divided into the following categories:

- Simple sugars - these are monosaccharides often seen on food labels as glucose or fructose

- Double sugars (or disaccharides) - these are seen on labels as sucrose (sugar), maltose, dextrose or lactose and are all a type of milk sugar

- Complex sugars (or polysaccharides) - which are starches and are found in grains, lentils, beans, potatoes and vegetables. All these sugars are broken down into glucose

Good sources of complex carbohydrate

- Wholewheat pasta

- Wholewheat bread

- High-fibre breakfast cereals

- Oats

- Root vegetables

- Beans and pulses

- Fruit

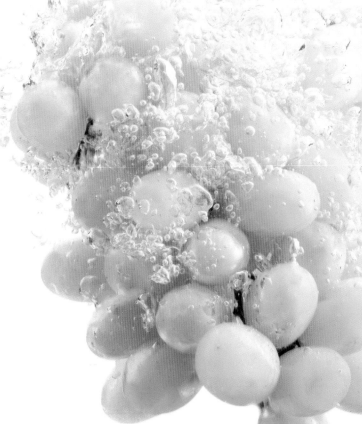

Types of carbohydrates to limit

- Sugar

- Chocolate

- Biscuits

- Soft, sugary drinks

- Jam, honey

- White bread

- White rice

- Crisps

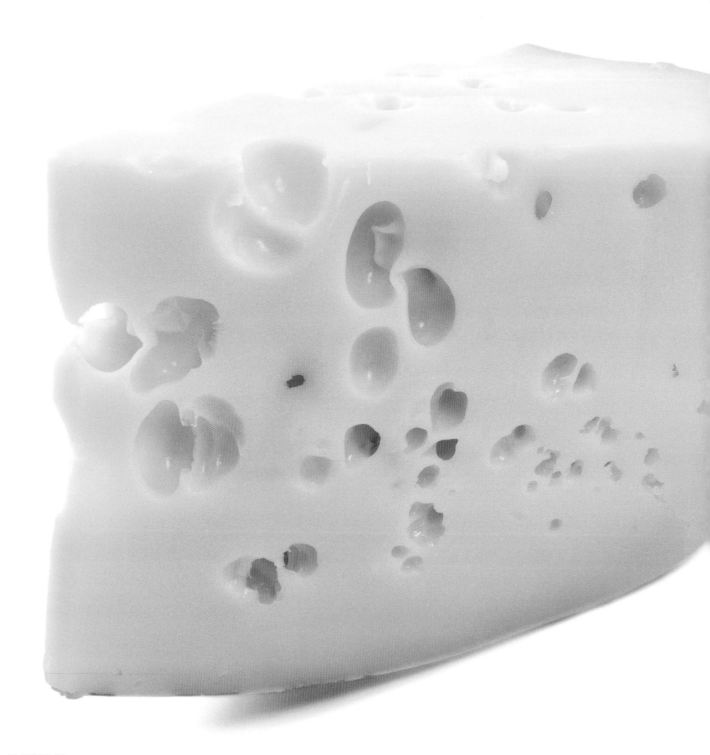

~ Protein ~

What does it do?

It is essential for growth and development, cell maintenance, the repair of muscles and the regulation of all body functions. Protein makes up every part of our skin, hair, nails, bone, tendons and muscles. It is also the main component of hormones such as insulin, which is needed to help control blood sugar levels, and calcitonin, which maintains levels of calcium in the bones (and therefore helps to protect against osteoporosis).

One of the most important roles of protein is to form haemoglobin, which carries oxygen to all the cells in the body to maintain energy levels and stamina. Enzymes, which act as the catalyst for many important bodily functions, are also made up of protein. Digestive enzymes help break down the food we eat and a protein deficiency may contribute to bloating, bad breath, constipation or low energy levels.

What is it?

Protein is made up of small building blocks called amino acids. When protein is broken down by digestion, it results in 22 known amino acids. Eight are essential; the body cannot manufacture them, the rest are non-essential and can be manufactured by the body with sound nutrition.

What's the best source of protein?

It is important to get protein from as wide a range of foods as possible to ensure you get all 22 amino acids. Foods that include no protein include vegetables, nut oils and refined sugar. The best sources of protein are Quorn, skinless poultry, fish, very lean meat, tofu, peas and beans, dairy products, eggs, milk and cheese.

Soya milk is also excellent. Low in saturated fat and high in unsaturated fat, soya milk has the added benefit of being high in calcium and phytoestrogens, which may protect against osteoporosis and menopausal symptoms such as hot flushes.

How much do I need?

In the past it was suggested that only 15% of daily calories should come from protein. However, latest research suggests that eating as much as 25-30% of daily calories from low-fat sources may be beneficial. While a high protein diet can lead to weight loss, it rarely leads to long-term fat loss. Eating too many sources of high-fat protein may lead to toxicity (when the body is unable to rid itself of all the toxins from food), which can result in sluggishness and bad skin.

A rough guideline is to eat no more than a hand-size portion of protein for lunch and dinner. For breakfast, try a smoothie made with soya milk and fruit, porridge or an oat-based cereal. A protein-based breakfast kick-starts your metabolism, encouraging the release of energy from fat.

Protein is believed to play a part in controlling appetite and encouraging the activity of a hormone called glucagon, which stimulates the release of glucose into the blood by breaking down glycogen (the body's store of carbohydrates). What this means is that your body stores less fat and the extra glucose in your bloodstream gives you more energy. A protein-rich lunch can also help to counter the 4pm chocolate run! But if you're still getting cravings, try eating nuts to keep your energy levels up.

~ Fats ~

What do they do?

Fats come in many forms, some of which are essential for forming cell walls, growth, sexual reproduction and maintaining the skin. Fat carries important vitamins such as A, D, E and K and provides twice as much energy as carbohydrates.

Without sufficient essential fats, which are vital to the body's metabolism, energy may decease and weight gain may increase.

Lastly, fats provide texture and flavour in food making it more palatable, and they help to give a feeling of fullness (the satiety value) after a meal.

What are they?

There are two types of 'good' essential (polyunsaturated) fats: Omega 3 and Omega 6. Omega 3 fats are found in oily fish such as herring, mackerel, salmon and tuna, as well as nuts, such as almonds, and seeds, such as linseed and pumpkin. Omega 6 fats are found in sunflower seeds and oil, sesame seeds and evening primrose oil.

Omega 6 oils are more widely used than Omega 3 and for this reason Omega 3 deficiency is fairly common. Symptoms may include dry skin, low energy, weight gain and poor concentration. Add seeds to your morning cereal or smoothies to boost your intake of essential fats, or scatter on to the top of soups, in with salads or into yoghurt. Hemp seeds, which are available in capsule form, are the best source of both fats.

- Monounsaturated fat (min. 35-45gms a day) - liquid at room temperature. Found in olive oil, rapeseed oil, fresh olives, nuts, avocados, eggs, fish, dairy products etc.

- Polyunsaturated fat (min. 18-25gms a day) - liquid at room temperature. Found in vegetable oils and most nuts, oily fish (salmon, mackerel, herring, sardines, tuna and trout), sunflower margarine and mayonnaise. These help to lower LDL (low density lipoproteins) blood cholesterol. They contain a high level of essential fatty acids (EFAs) that the body cannot produce and can therefore only be provided by your diet. This oil should not be used for cooking because it becomes oxidised when heated and this can actually damage the body by producing free radicals.

- Saturated fat (max. 25-30gms a day) - usually solid at room temperature. Found in animal produce such as meat, cheese, cream, suet, butter and lard, chocolate, cakes, crisps and biscuits etc. Causes a high level of LDL blood cholesterol that is a major factor in the incidence of heart disease, obesity and cancer.

- Trans fats (max. 2-4gms a day) - hydrogenated in food processing and hard at room temperature. This is the only fat that raises the bad LDL cholesterol and lowers the good HDL (high density lipoproteins) cholesterol. Found in cooking fats, mass-produced cakes etc, and take-away foods such as fish and chips. In modern food production, such fats are prevalent in mass produced, processed foods. They are listed as trans fats or hydrogenated vegetable oils and should be avoided at all costs.

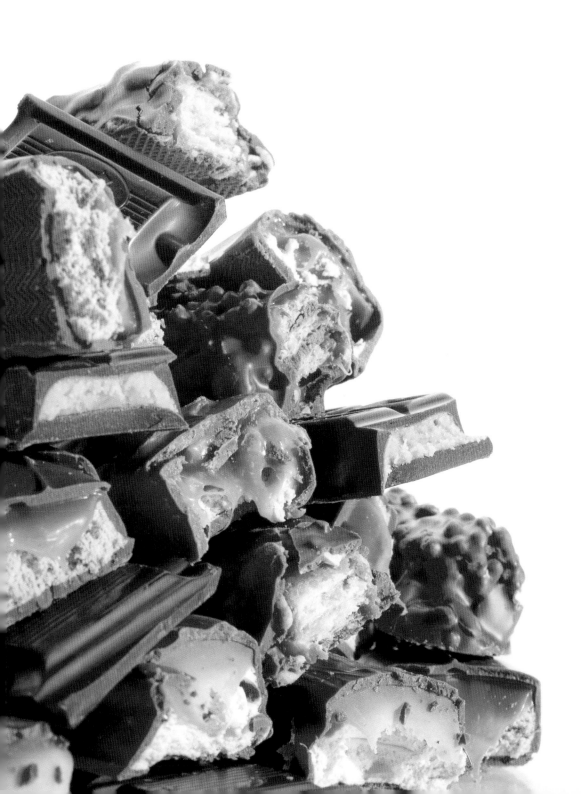

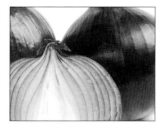

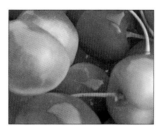

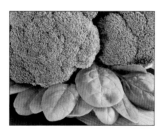

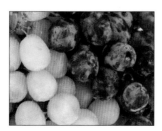

Vitamins and minerals are frequently referred to as the micronutrients in contrast to fats, proteins and carbohydrates, which are referred to as macronutrients. The reason for this is related to the amounts needed by the body. Macronutrients are required in weights that are easily measured by ordinary kitchen scales; despite being essential, micronutrients are only required in very small amounts.

The condition of the skin is often a sign of how healthy the body's cells are overall. They depend on supplies of zinc, magnesium, iron and other minerals.

By ensuring you eat a balanced and varied diet you will most certainly get all of the necessary vitamins and minerals your body needs to function effectively. Different sources of carbohydrate, types of protein, lots of different vegetables, salads and fruits not only prevent boredom in a diet, they also ensure you get all of the micronutrients you need. Different foods will provide you with different nutrients.

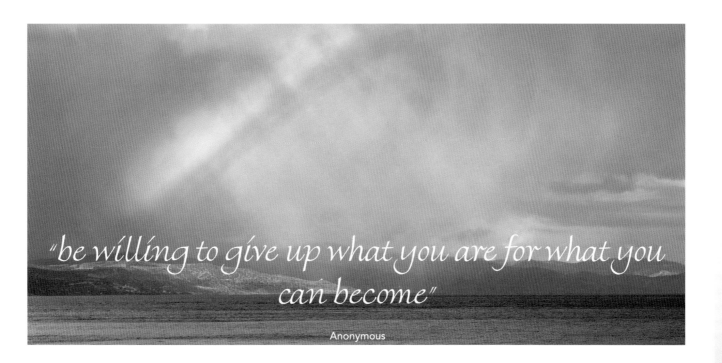

"be willing to give up what you are for what you can become"

Anonymous

~ *Water* ~

In short, it's vital, and without it our bodies wouldn't function. Water is as valuable to us as energy - 70% of the body is water and it is vital to life.

Inadequate water consumption plays a huge part in low energy levels and feeling drained all the time. Insufficient fluid intake can compromise the body's eliminatory process, something that then undermines the immune function and hormone balance. Water is an essential nutrient that's involved in every function of the body - anything from transporting nutrients and waste products in and out of cells, to maintaining a proper body temperature. We all need to ensure we drink approximately 1–1½ litres of water each day, increasing when exercising or to compensate for eating or drinking stimulants.

There will no doubt be relief to learn that drinking water is not the only way of increasing the fluid intake. Fruit and vegetables consist of around 90% water, and they supply it in a form that is very easy for the body to use. At the same time, they provide a high percentage of vitamins and minerals. The seed vegetables appear to be the most effective (peas, corn, broad beans, broccoli, runner beans etc). These also provide good levels of protein and help neutralise excess acidity, which can lead to the loss of minerals, including calcium.

Four pieces of fruit and four vegetables amount to approximately 1kg, which would equal roughly 1 litre of water. The other litre could consist of diluted juices, herb and fruit teas, in particular fennel, dandelion, ginger and peppermint.

Food for thought - for women aged 20-40

- Drink at least 1–1½ litres each day

- Eat at least 5 portions of fresh fruit and vegetables each day

- Drink no more than 4-5 cups of tea, coffee or cola daily

- Keep alcohol intake to 14 units a week (1 unit = a small glass of wine, measure of spirit or half a pint of beer or lager)

- Always eat a healthy breakfast – this can be a smoothie

- Eat oily fish at least 3 times a week

- Cut down on highly processed and ready-made food

- Try to restrict red meat to 2-3 times a week

- Remove the salt cellar from the table

- Use vegetable and olive oil rather than animals fats and butter where possible

Food for thought - for women aged 50-70

- Eat small meals more frequently

- Cut down on refined sugar, tea, coffee, alcohol and processed foods

- Eat a diet rich in soya and other foods rich in phytoestrogens

- Have at least 8 glasses of water each day

- Try to eat 6 servings of bread, rice, fortified cereals or pasta daily

- Avoid yo-yo dieting at all costs

- Eat 5 portions of fresh fruit and vegetables each day

- Eat fats, oils and sweets sparingly

- Take supplements of calcium and a multi-vitamin to protect against deficiencies

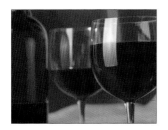
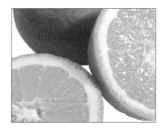
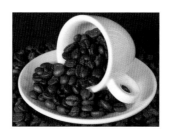
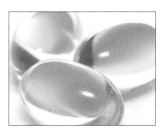

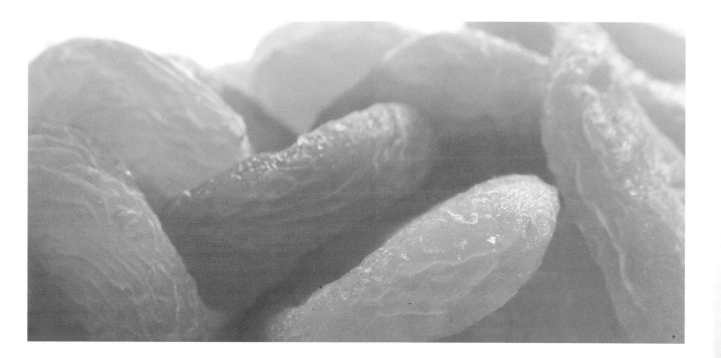

Nutrition for Glowing Skin

The most common agents affecting the skin's integrity are the free radicals that attack it, both externally from cigarette smoke, pollution and UV light, and internally from a diet low in essential nutrients and high in hydrogenated fats, trans-fatty acids, fried food, barbequed food and highly processed food. Free radicals are produced during the body's normal metabolism process, and can generally be managed by our normal elimination processes. However, if excess free radicals occur, or there is an absence of antioxidants, damage to the skin can occur.

A diet rich in antioxidants, along with a lifestyle that reduces the level of free radicals, will help to combat the ageing and damaging effects of these sad little atoms. The following are some fabulous antioxidant foods.

- Vitamin A - found in the diet in two basic forms, Beta Carotene and Retinol.

- Beta Carotene - most orange, yellow and dark green produce contains beta carotene, including cantaloupe melons, apricots, peppers, pumpkins, carrots, swedes, turnips, parsley, squash, sweet potatoes and green leafy vegetables.

- Retinol - found in animal foods such as lambs liver, oily fish, fish oil supplements, eggs and cheese.

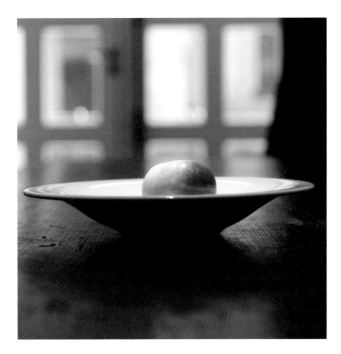

~ Vitamin C ~

Ascorbate, Ascorbic Acid

Vital for fighting infection, for wound healing and for the formation of collagen, often referred to as the cement that holds the skin together. Collagen degeneration can be linked to a lack of vitamin C and when the elasticity of collagen collapses, skin sags and ages very quickly. As well as this, vitamin C has hundreds of other biochemical tasks. It reduces the risk of arterial damage and cardiovascular disease, balances blood cholesterol, protects against stress, reduces allergic reactions and is needed for energy production. Vitamin C is water-soluble; the body needs a daily supply because water-soluble nutrients are not stored by the body's system.

Vitamin C is found in:

- Kiwi fruits (there is twice as much vitamin C in a single kiwi as in a large orange)

- Apricots, grapefruit, cranberries, mango, blackcurrants, acerola cherries, kumquats, guava, papaya and strawberries

- Tomatoes, green leafy vegetables, peas, cauliflower, green and red peppers

- Jacket potatoes

Skin symptoms of vitamin C shortage include:

- Easy bruising

- Cuts that won't heal

- Broken capillaries

- Poor immunity

~ Vitamin A ~

A lack of vitamin A damages cell membranes causing new cells to die off before they have a chance to reach the surface, blocking the pores and preventing lubrication of the skin. Vitamin A also enhances the activity of EFAs, in particular gamma linolenic acid (GLA). It works closely with zinc to support the immune function and helps to transport other life-sustaining nutrients to the cells.

Skin symptoms of vitamin A shortage include:

- Dry, rough, scaly skin

- Inflamed eyelids

- Spots, pimples, boils

- Recurring skin infections

- Sore, burning, itchy eyes (in the absence of poor sleep and external irritants)

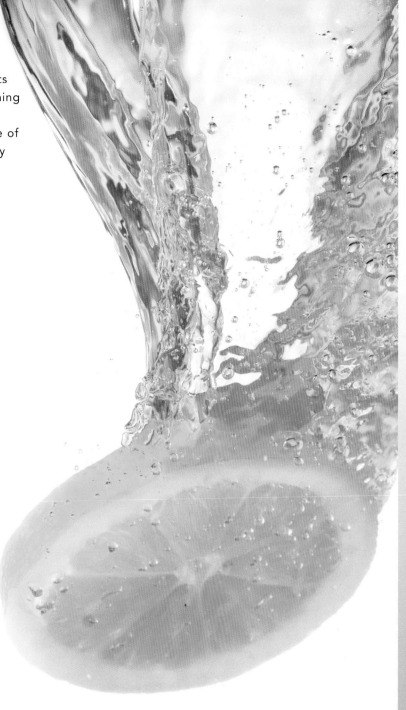

~ Bioflavonoids ~

Bioflavonoids increase the potency of antioxidants and maintain cell membranes, especially those lining blood vessels and collagen. They are found with vitamin C in plant foods and are the major source of their red and blue pigments (the carotenes supply the majority of orange, dark green and yellow colour).

Bioflavonoids are found in:

- White rind of citrus fruits (particularly lemons)

- Vegetables

- Buckwheat

- Honey

- Fresh apricots

- Blackcurrants

- Beetroot

- Broccoli

~ Vitamin E ~

Tocopherol

Amongst other things, vitamin E is the vitamin for reducing scarring following an accident or surgery. It can also reduce the prominence of old scars if applied topically on a regular basis, and has been used to help burn victims. Vitamin E is known to prolong cell life, improve skin quality and hasten wound healing.

Vitamin E is found in:

- Wheatgerm oil*, wheatgerm,
- Soybean oil, olive oil
- Wholegrains (especially brown rice)
- Egg yolk
- Liver
- Nuts (particularly almonds and walnuts)
- Sprouted grains
- Green vegetables
- Sunflower seeds and sunflower oil

Extra vitamin E is helpful where there is:

- Dry skin and also oily skin
- Scarring
- Eczema
- Acne
- Psoriasis
- Stretch marks
- Easy bruising
- Stress
- Hormonal imbalances

*wheatgerm is often suggested as a rich source of vitamin E but it has a very short shelf life and is prone to rapid rancidity once opened

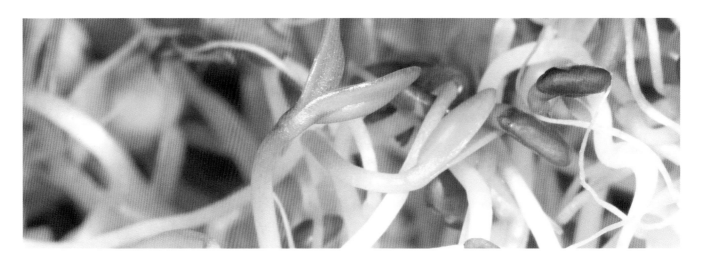

~ Manganese ~

Manganese is an essential trace element that is necessary for the normal functioning of the brain, and is effective in the treatment of many nervous disorders. Our understanding of manganese is still incomplete due to research into this important trace element remaining in its infancy. It may prove to be one of the most important nutrients in human pathology.

Sources include:

- Cereals

- Black tea

- Green leaf vegetables

- Rice bran

- Wholewheat bread

- Legumes

- Ginger and cloves

- Nuts

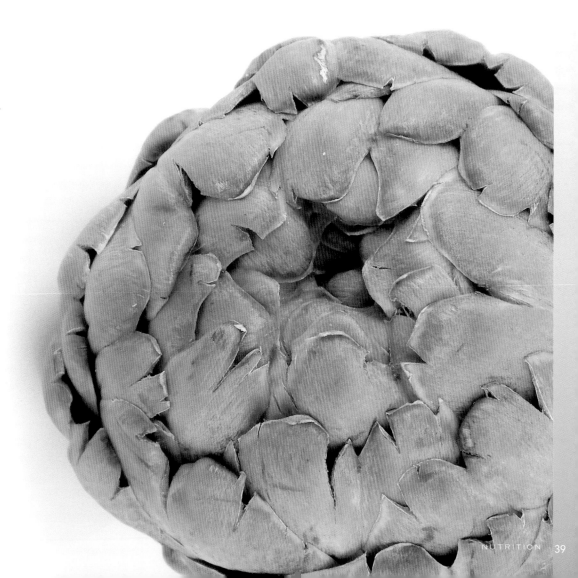

~ Selenium ~

Selenium is a trace element and is needed in tiny amounts. It is an excellent antioxidant, provides protection against free radical activity and pollution, and supports the immune function. It works in synergy with vitamins C and E.

Selenium is found in:

- Brazil nuts and cashews

- Molasses

- Bran

- Onions and tomatoes

- Soybeans

- Tuna and seafood

- Meat and kidneys

- Wholegrains (brown rice)

Selenium is also found in many vegetables but this varies depending upon the amount of selenium present in the soil where the crop was grown.

Selenium deficiency signs include:

- Dry, flaking skin

- Poor wound healing

- Stiff, painful joints

- Poor immunity

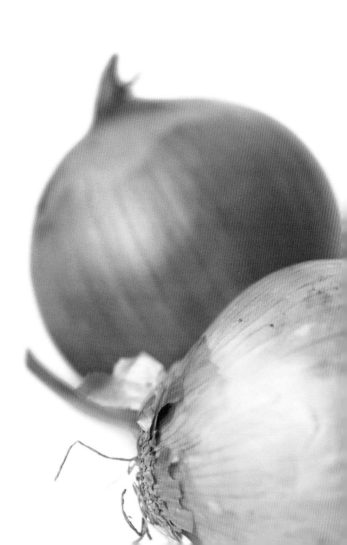

Zinc ~

The benefits that zinc imparts to the skin should not be underestimated. Without zinc, vitamin A cannot be properly used. Zinc is vital for growth and repair, for wound healing, strengthening the immune system, balancing insulin production as well as for helping other hormones. Healthy growth and repair of cells also depend on zinc in the diet.

Zinc is found in:

- Seafood, in particular oysters, and fish

- Popcorn

- Pumpkin seeds

- Wheatgerm

- Meat

- Eggs

Zinc deficiency signs include:

- Excessively dry or excessively oily skin

- Slow wound healing

- Acne

- Persistent infections

- White marks on the fingernails

- Poor digestion

- Loss of taste or smell

- Poor appetite

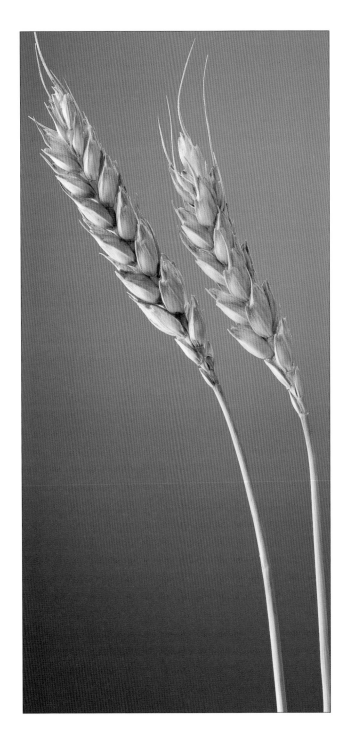

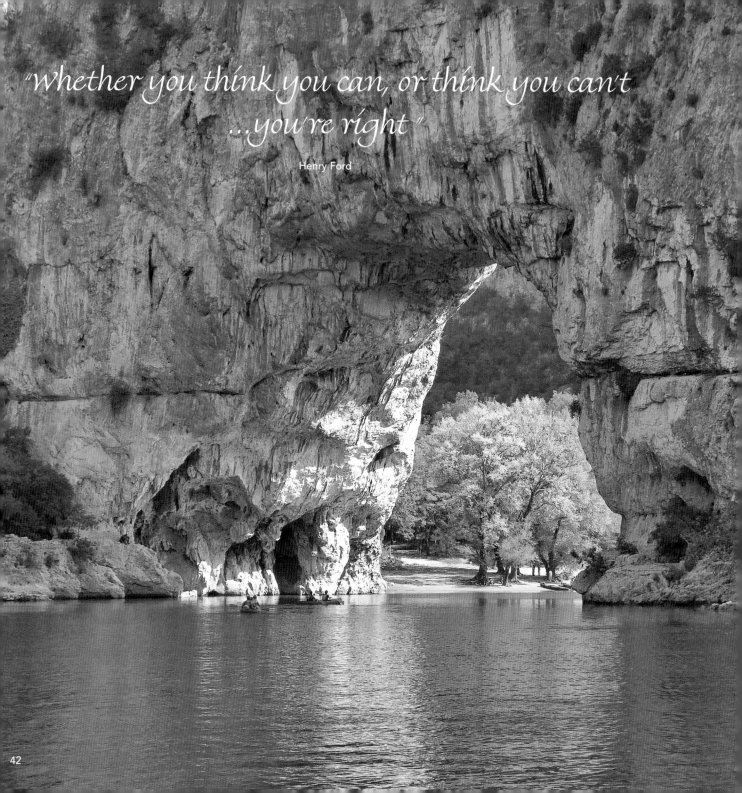

"whether you think you can, or think you can't
...you're right"

Henry Ford

EXERCISE

Exercise is now widely acknowledged as playing an integral role in our physical, mental and spiritual health, and it doesn't need to be the sweat and tears of the 'feel the burn' approach that fill most of us with dread. Clients know that we all need to take more physical exercise, and eat more healthily, but the pressure from the perception of how much exercise is needed to make a difference can stop many in their tracks. Helping clients to see how little you can get away with, whilst still enjoying the benefits of healthy skin and increased energy, can be enough to get them motivated to start.

Daily activity lifts mood, reduces anxiety and depression, dissipates negative stress, helps to detoxify the body and helps it shed old and unwanted dead skin cells. When we exercise, the blood and lymph flow are increased, which means freshly oxygenated blood is drawn to the surface of the skin, bringing with it fresh nutrients and improved removal of waste products. This means skin tone is improved, the ageing process is slowed down and muscle strength and lean body mass is improved, helping to prevent sagging!

Exercise is not confined to high aerobic workouts that get many of us panting, hot and sweaty. It is as much about gentle aerobics, keep fit classes, yoga, t'ai chi, cycling, walking, swimming, dancing, stretching and deep breathing that help enhance our mental and spiritual well-being. One thing is for sure: exercise should and must become an integral part of our daily routine. Encouraging clients to exercise can be tough but your encouragement for them to get started can bring about immediate benefits, especially to stressed clients.

Perhaps seeing the gym as a get-away zone, or walking the dog as chill-out time can be enough to gain a much needed perspective on the pressures of daily life. I once saw a quote that 'everyone should take their dog for walk, even if they don't have one'. Mine have certainly been the best motivation to move away from the computer or resist the lure of my pillow in the morning!

This section is not aiming to make fitness instructors or personal trainers of all skincare therapists. But it is intended to be thought-provoking and informative about some of the benefits of taking more regular exercise.

Exercise is the most effective anti-ageing pill ever discovered.

National Institute of Health

- A full 95% of people who follow a weight reducing diet will, after a three-year period, at best regain every ounce of the weight they have lost, and at worst end up weighing more than when they began (and feel tons worse psychologically).

- 70% of the body is made up of water, and it is very easy to lose 10lbs of water within several days. Dehydration is positively harmful and is nothing to do with real weight loss.

- It's not how much an individual weighs but how much fat they're carrying around that makes the difference to their well-being, health and body shape. To lose fat, aim at slow and steady weight loss, no more than 1- 2lbs a week.

- If people lose more fat than this, the body will think it is being starved to death, and its very powerful defences against starvation start to kick in. The most important of these defences is a reduction in the body's metabolic rate. This means the body will make less energy (leading to fatigue and lethargy) and produce less heat (causing greater sensitivity to cold).

- If weight loss is achieved using diet alone, at least 25-30% of the weight being shed is not fat but water, muscle and other lean tissue. And the faster the weight is lost (over 2lbs of weight a week), the less of it will be fat. This is a disaster for long-term weight loss as muscle tissue is 5 times more metabolically active than fat tissue.

- Metabolically active means it requires a lot of calories for maintenance, even in its resting state. It's estimated that 500g of muscle burns 75 calories a day, whereas 500g (1lb) of fat uses up only around 8 calories.

- To remove excess fat effectively, we need to increase our level of activity and so increase energy output. Exercise, on its own without dieting, doesn't actually help promote much weight loss; running a mile only burns around 300 calories!

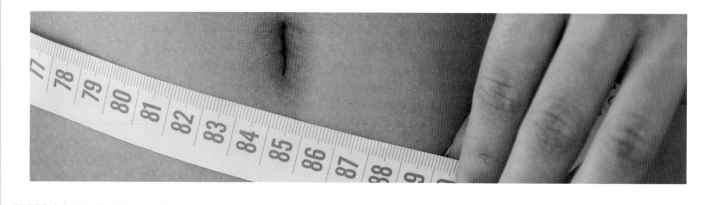

Aerobic exercise metabolises calories and raises the metabolic rate. The heart rate needs to be raised to 55-90% of a person's maximum heart rate for 20-30 minutes three times a week. The metabolic rate will be raised for 24 hours after exercising.

Resistance, or weight training, builds muscle mass. Aerobic exercise may burn calories, but it does not prevent muscle loss. If muscle is lost, the most metabolically active part of your body is lost. Resistance training needs to be carried out 2-3 times a week for between 20 and 30 minutes.

Since the amount of fat people carry is a far more important statistic than their weight, encourage clients not to use the scales as the only means of monitoring progress. Encouragement in the early days is likely to come from a reduction of 'vital statistics' rather than a loss of weight – so get the tape measure out!

Finally, good nutrition is very important for fat loss, and focusing on health and health-promoting foods is far more productive than focusing on fat loss and denial of favourite foods. Adopting a wholefood diet, reducing and avoiding saturated fats, sugar, salt, additives, preservatives and refined foods, needs to become a lifestyle change.

Move more, sit less...

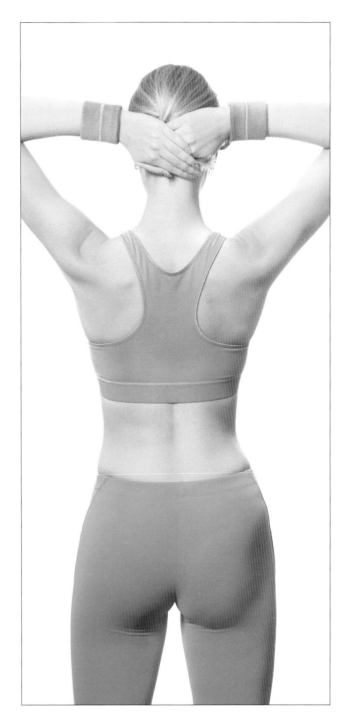

- Sensations of hunger can result from being on a diet or from malnourishment. Such clients may not be getting enough minerals and/or vitamins, or there might be an imbalance of carbohydrates, proteins and fats.

- Whatever the particular deficiency or imbalance, the body's metabolism will register the shortage, and the signal it is likely to be sending to the brain is 'eat more', resulting in a feeling of hunger. For example, if the body is unable to maintain proper metabolic balances because of a deficiency of, say, chromium, blood sugar will fluctuate greatly, causing fat deposition when it rises and hunger as it falls.

- Eating more, better quality foods (those relieved of their chemical load but bursting with micronutrients, antioxidants and phytochemicals) will also help to eliminate the body's need to manufacture fat.

- This is due to another function of fat, which is that of toxin storage. Many of the substances in our environment are poisonous, and the vast majority of these are fat-soluble (preservatives, additives, coffee, alcohol, fats and so on). If the body is unable to metabolise and remove these materials, they tend to become stored away in the fatty tissue.

- The body may even manufacture fat especially for the storage of dangerous substances. Due to the relatively low metabolism of fatty tissue, once toxins are stored here they are likely to remain undisturbed; the body becomes very reluctant to have them circulate again.

- This fat becomes most persistent. Further fat tends to get dumped in these places because the metabolism has 'learned' to do this with a wider range of substances it doesn't like.

- If the weight problem is caused by fat retention to protect against toxins, it will become apparent as individuals lose weight; they will begin to experience some of the symptoms of detoxification, such as a furry tongue, headaches, fever, rash and tiredness. For this reason, it may be necessary to carry out a gentle detoxification programme.

- Eat the correct balance of protein, carbohydrate and fat, and eat when genuinely hungry rather than just for comfort.

- Stop eating when feeling full and not to clear the plate.

- Encourage the client to understand that when they eat, they eat. When they have a meal don't drive, walk, watch the TV or read - just enjoy the food.

- Aim to get the client's body into hormonal balance so that the controlled burning of excess fat will maintain them as a naturally slim person. And slow down. Most overweight people gobble and miss the brain's satiety cues. If it helps, encourage clients to put their knife and fork down between mouthfuls.

- Fill the shopping trolley with label-free foods - in other words, fruit and vegetables!

- A good idea is for clients to keep a diary for a week about how foods make them feel 20 minutes or 2 hours after they have eaten. Get clients to choose foods that make them feel alert and energised, not tired and bloated.

- For clients new to exercise, try getting them to put 10p into a jar every time they do 15 minutes' continuous exercise. Their goal is to bank 3-4 coins a day. Then they can splash out on a reward when they've reached their goal.

- It helps to try to plan a week's menus in advance. It's not just what people eat each day but how the diet stacks up over time that causes the problems (or solves them!).

- If you've got a client who is prone to snacking, before they succumb ask them to spend 10 minutes evaluating what they really need. It could be that they are 'hungry' for sex, companionship or even fresh air. Avoid using food as a substitute.

- Every 30 minutes, aim to stand up and move around for 5 minutes non-stop.

Prevent an obsession with food, which itself will cause stress and a slowing down of metabolism.

The greatest gift you will ever receive is the gift of loving and believing in yourself. Guard this with your life. It is the only thing that will ever truly be yours.

Tiffany Loren Rowe

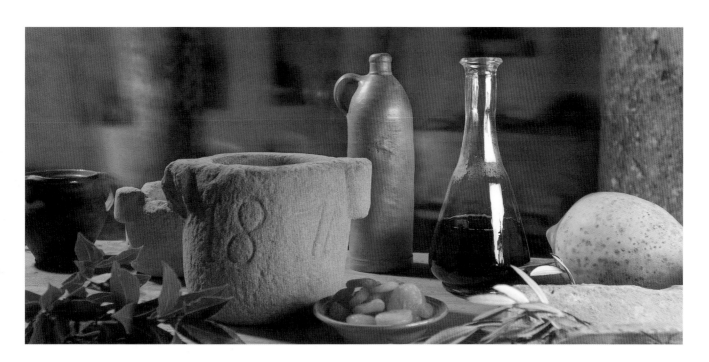

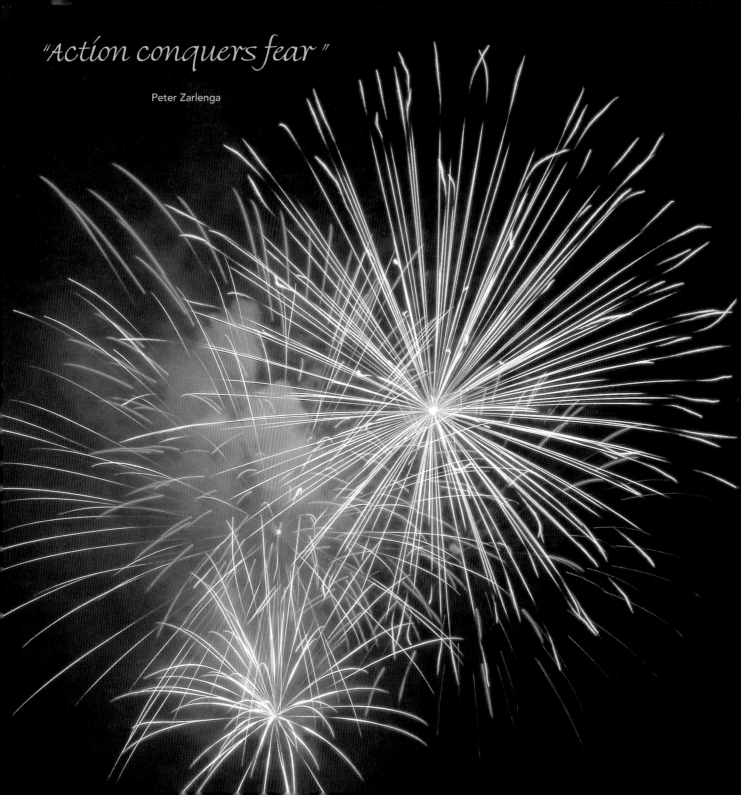

"Action conquers fear"

Peter Zarlenga

STRESS

The aim of this chapter is to familiarise you with some recognisable symptoms that clients may present with when experiencing high or sustained levels of stress. It is helpful to hold these in mind when working holistically and recognising the unspoken with your clients. This knowledge should help inform your thinking when deciding upon the right treatment plan or appropriate home care advice you offer your client.

Stress has been compared to love or electricity - it's an unmistakable experience but difficult to define!

The following is a selection of definitions of what is meant by this word, 'stress'. The HSE (Health & Safety Executive) define it as 'the adverse reaction people have to excessive pressure or other types of demand placed on them'. A simpler option is to think of it as 'the internalisation of pressure, where it exceeds your ability to cope'. However, the following definition is my favourite: 'the confusion created when one's mind overrides the body's basic desire to choke the living daylights out of someone who desperately needs it'!

The figure here, 'The Pressure Curve', shows what we mean by this.

- If the amount of pressure is not high enough, we do not feel the need to respond and so performance is likely to be down.

- Get the pressure 'right' and we are triggered to respond in the most effective way - and will operate at our 'optimal performance' level.

- Moving along towards the end, the pressure levels increase and when this is too much the response is what most people think of as the classic stress problem, 'burn out'.

- This rarely just 'happens' suddenly. The pressures build up, the symptoms will become more and more obvious, the physiological and behavioural clues will be more noticeable.

- If the situation does not change, and the pressure becomes more unmanageable, the person who is at this end will probably start to become ill as the body sends out signals to say it needs to protect itself against this burn-out.

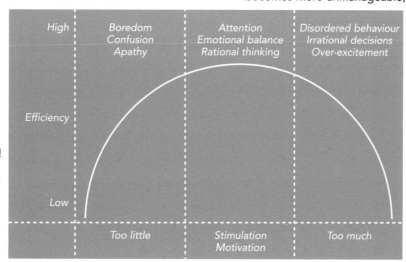

~ Effects of stress on industry ~

The effects of stress have a huge cost on industry and is one of the biggest underlying risk factors within an organisation. Let us start by looking at some hard-nosed numbers (based on the UK.)

- The CBI estimates that there is a cost of £4bn per annum to industry as a direct result of stress-related absence.

- This figure can rise to over £7bn when you consider the loss of productivity.

- A recent survey by the HSE indicated over 550,000 cases of absence as a result of stress, depression and anxiety.

- A further 66,000 were absent with heart problems as a result of stress.

- There was a loss of nearly 13m working days in total.

- The average absence was 28.5 days for stress-related issues.

- 1 in 5 believes that their job is extremely or very stressful - that is 5 million people!

- Up to 40% of absence is related to stress.

- When stressed, performance can be reduced by up to 70%.

- The CIPD (Chartered Institute of Personnel and Development) estimate that stress costs industry £522 per employee.

We each interpret stress in different ways. What one of us may shrug off, another will think of as a crisis and vice versa. These stresses can come from many different sources - anything from personal relationships, financial pressures, illness, environmental stresses such as travelling to work (think of the poor individuals travelling into central London after the terrorist attacks in 2005), and also the stress we put on ourselves through unrealistic expectations and an obsession with material goods.

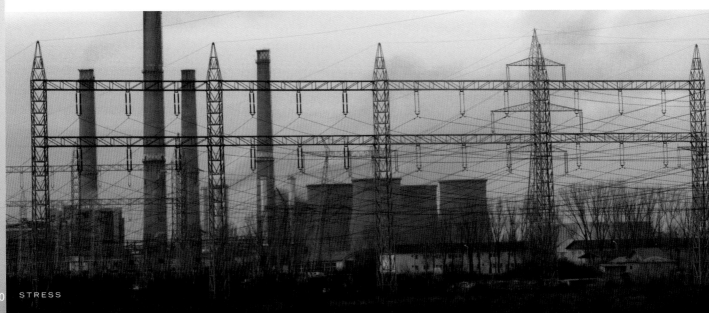

~ Physiological effects of stress ~

The way our bodies respond to stress was described in the 1930s by two American doctors, Walter B Cannon and Hans Seyle. They found the first reaction is what is known as the 'flight or fight' response, which activates the body's protective mechanism to either confront stress or avoid it. Initially this response alerts us to danger and provides the strength, speed and stamina needed for survival.

The stress response is controlled by the endocrine (hormone) system. Any unusual demand on the physical and mental resources stimulates the hypothalamus, pituitary and adrenal glands to secrete hormones (adrenalin, cortisol, testosterone and thyroxin) directly into the blood stream. These produce a variety of physical responses:

- Dilated pupils

- Increased perspiration

- Increased heart rate and blood pressure

- Rapid breathing

- Muscle tension

- Increased blood flow to the brain, heart and muscles

- Reduced blood flow to the skin and digestive tract

- Increased mental awareness and sensitivity

- Increased release of blood sugar

- A rise in platelets and blood clotting factors

These responses are life-saving for short-term, stressful situations - like being chased by a bull - but fighting or running away are rarely appropriate responses to modern-day stressful situations. Under long-term or chronic stress, our bodies remain in a constant heightened state, with the gradual on-set of health problems, some of which are listed on the following page.

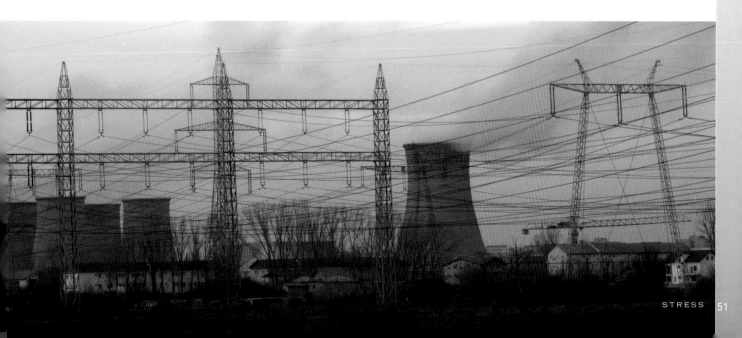

Cardio-vascular disease

- High blood pressure

- Arteriosclerosis (thickening of the artery wall)

- Angina

- Stroke

- Heart failure

Immune system:

- Low resistance to colds and general infections

- Cold sores

- Cancer

Skin complaints:

- Acne

- Spots/skin breakouts

- Eczema

- Psoriasis

- Sallow complexion

Digestive system:

- IBS

- Ulcers

- Constipation/diarrhoea

- Indigestion

- Heartburn

~ Psychological reactions to stress~

The way we react to stress is as individual as we are, and consequently how we respond to stress is vital. We all need a certain amount of stress to function, but when stress levels reach extremes and we can no longer deal with it, it becomes a problem. Not dealing with our stress levels can lead to many symptoms and diseases as already mentioned, along with asthma, diabetes, migraine, headaches, fatigue, insomnia and depression. So try to help clients to reframe how they respond to different circumstances. Stress will either help or hinder us depending on how we react to it.

The psychological or emotional signs of stress can be:

- Mood swings

- Being abrasive or hostile (when normally passive and friendly)

- Becoming depressed

- Over anxious

- Panic attacks

- Sudden levels of disorganisation

- Lethargy or general lack of interest

- Negative self-introspection

- Poor judgement

- Confusion

None of these signs are conclusive but certainly warrant some attention by your client.

> *Spiral Effects of Constant Stress*

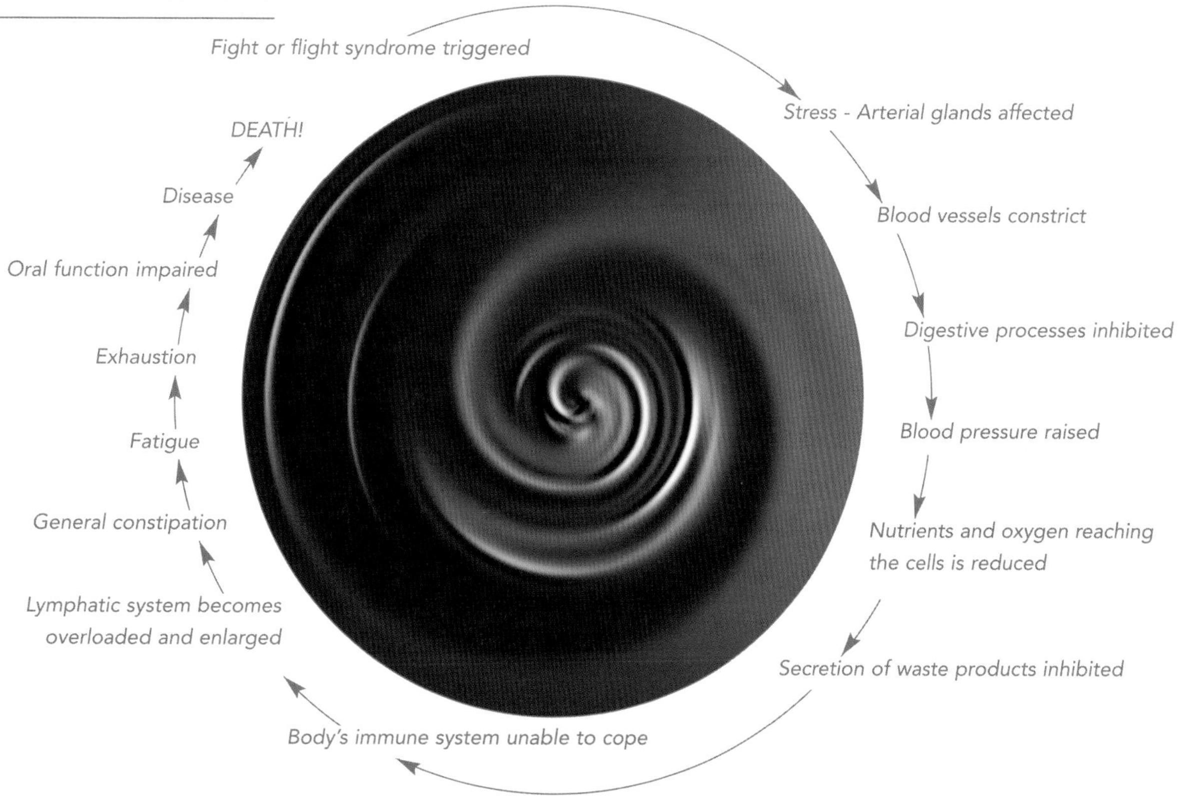

Fight or flight syndrome triggered

DEATH!

Stress - Arterial glands affected

Disease

Oral function impaired

Blood vessels constrict

Exhaustion

Digestive processes inhibited

Fatigue

Blood pressure raised

General constipation

Nutrients and oxygen reaching the cells is reduced

Lymphatic system becomes overloaded and enlarged

Secretion of waste products inhibited

Body's immune system unable to cope

~ Coping strategies~

When the body is under stress, particularly long-term (chronic) stress, it needs careful handling nutritionally in order both to minimise the stress and ensure that nutrient requirements are met. Stress tends to deplete the body of certain vital vitamins and minerals, and anyone under long-term stress should either be extra careful to incorporate plenty of these into the diet by eating the right foods, or should take good quality supplements.

The vitamin B group is largely responsible for the smooth running of the nervous system and, as the B group is water-soluble and cannot be stored in the body for very long, chronic stress will soon severely deplete it.

The same applies to vitamin C, which most experts believe a stressed person will need in much greater quantities than the RNI of 40mg a day - 200mg is probably more appropriate.

Zinc (which helps strengthen the immune system, wound healing and so on) and Magnesium (which is excreted in greater amounts when under stress) may need to be supplemented, or zinc- and magnesium-rich foods scrupulously incorporated into the diet. Great nutritional sources of zinc include wheatgerm, calves liver, poppy seeds, oysters, Quorn, pine nuts and All Bran. For magnesium, include lots of cocoa powder, sunflower seeds, Brazil nuts, sesame seeds and cashew nuts.

Bodies depleted of vitamins B and C and zinc are also at increased risk of getting almost constant infections, cold sores, dry, rough, scaly skin, broken capillaries and so on, because these are the nutrients that help protect against these symptoms.

Also take into consideration that many of your

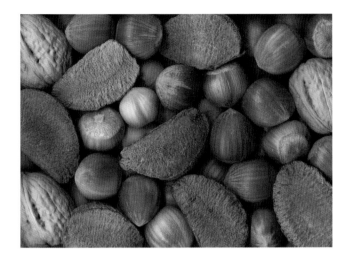

stressed clients may turn to alcohol and smoking for relief. Both of these make the nutritional problems worse as both, like stress, also deplete the body of B and C vitamins and can hinder the absorption of many others. Remember not to judge your clients' choices but work 'with the given'. Encourage them to boost their nutrient intake through excellent nutrition. This may appear controversial: as I've described already, my own feeling about smoking is that if the fear of cancer isn't enough to motivate them to stop, then the depletion of a few vitamins and minerals, with the consequent skin problems, certainly won't shock them into giving up!

A great nutritional strategy to help tackle stress is to eat plenty of complex carbohydrates, such as pasta and whole grains, which will help the brain to calm down by helping to release the chemical serotonin. Chronic stress, and the higher levels of adrenalin it produces, raises the levels of fats and cholesterol in the blood. This can be a contributory factor in the increased risk of circulatory and heart disease.

Often when coping with high levels of stress, planning and preparing meals takes a low priority. However, as detailed already, this is when good nutrition is most important. The following is a summary of some of the recommendations you could incorporate into your aftercare advice for clients.

• A good start is to choose healthy snacks such as fruit over junk and fast foods.

• Drink plenty of water and replace tea and coffee with other, more gentle alternatives such as herbal, green or Rooibush teas.

• Make eating meals as relaxing as possible. Turn off the TV, put on some relaxing music and enjoy your food and your environment.

• Avoid eating on the move.

• Supplements of nutrients are very important at these times. A good multi-vitamin and mineral supplement is a vital part of stress management.

• Herbal remedies are of great value when helping clients to deal with stress. The appropriate herbs for each client will depend on their individual circumstances. You can, however, recommend that they see a herbalist or naturopath.

• Ginseng has become a popular stress management herb in recent times, as it enhances the ability to handle life.

• Relaxing at night is vital. Therefore, 'stimulating' TV or thriller novels need to be replaced with more relaxing alternatives.

• Herbal tea before bed can be relaxing, such as Rooibush (Redbush) or Chamomile.

• Burning relaxing essential oils will have a therapeutic effect, such as lavender, basil or petitgrain.

• Relax stress away in a warm bath with a few drops of essential oil.

• Spend time meditating to clear the mind.

• Focusing on deep breathing exercises will help to dissipate adrenalin.

• Exercise on a daily basis - brisk walking, swimming, yoga, t'ai chi and dancing for example.

• Relax, using massage, reflexology, facials, movies, books - create some 'me time'.

• Take up a hobby, something that absorbs the mind and needs concentration.

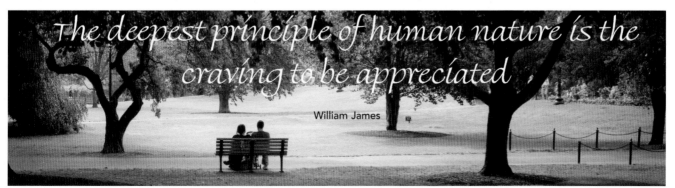

The deepest principle of human nature is the craving to be appreciated

William James

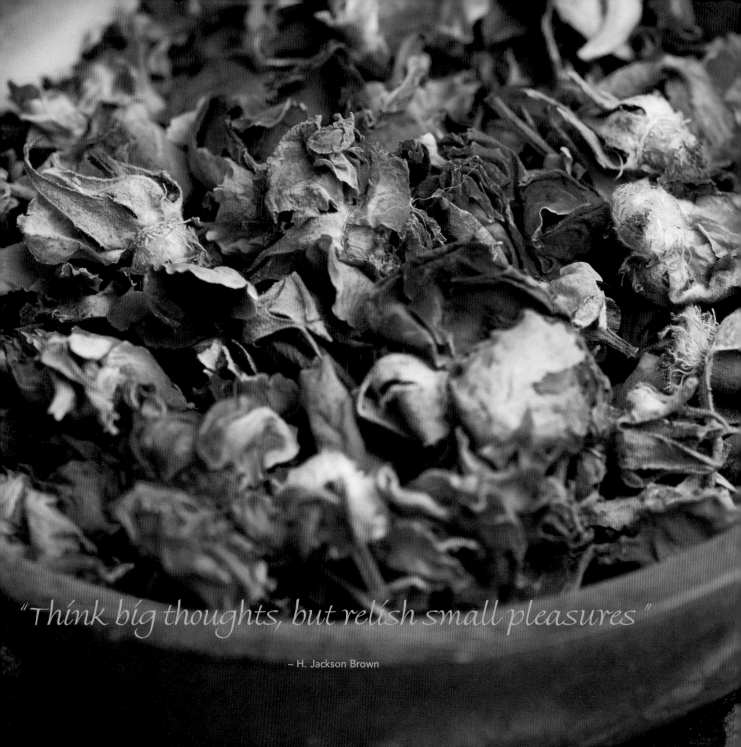

"Think big thoughts, but relish small pleasures"

– H. Jackson Brown

AROMATHERAPY

The objective of this chapter is to give you an understanding of the versatility and potency of essential oils, the various ways you and your clients can use them, and finally an overview of the oils that can assist in your role as the skincare therapist.

If you haven't yet felt the compulsive need to learn additional elements of holistic medicine then prepare for aromatherapy to give you the 'study bug' – the subject becomes addictive and once captivated you will find it difficult to stop, there is so much to learn!

Essential oils should never be used neat or taken internally unless specified by a qualified physician. Do make an effort to find a qualified aromatherapist in your area as they will be able to advise, prescribe and blend oils for you and your clients.

Introduction

The literal interpretation of the word aromatherapy is 'therapy through aroma'. In other words, the impact a particular smell has on us – negative or positive. Which is why we can now see household goods such as washing up liquid being marketed under the banner of aromatherapy – it doesn't mean it has any therapeutic benefit, it just means it smells nice.

It is no longer seen as 'folksy' with professional aromatherapy now available in spas, beauty salons, sports facilities and in some hairdressing products. Essential oils are now a conventional technique adopted in hospital maternity wards and natural health centres.

The healing powers of essential oils have been known for centuries but it has been the last two decades that have seen a remarkable renaissance in the practice and interest of aromatherapy. It is now one of the most popular complementary therapies available and is becoming increasingly accepted by GPs and midwives working in hospitals to be used alongside allopathic (or orthodox) medicine.

Although allopathic medicine is exciting in terms of the pace of success, and the scope of the pioneering work being done, many more people also want to know about preventative medicine which is drug-free, simple & safe. As mentioned in previous chapters, there is a tendency in modern medicine for a person to be treated as a symptom or disease rather than as a complete individual. In contrast, the use of essential oils by a qualified and practiced aromatherapist recognises that there is seldom one characteristic of an illness and time must be taken to discover these various parts.

As the world increases in speed, there is a need to slow down and notice the effect, both emotionally and physically, that the demands of this high-octane living has upon us. Taking the time to reflect and relax with an aromatherapy massage could provide the much needed solace a client needs.

My own philosophy has been about finding a balance between allopathic medicine and natural remedies. Care needs to be taken not to see natural remedies as a safe panacea: some natural remedies are highly dangerous. I would not want to see the progress of scientific advances being halted but I do want to provide information on essential oils, their versatile nature and how they can be used to benefit both the therapist and client in the arena of skincare.

The History of Essential Oils

Aromatherapy has at its roots the most ancient healing practices - possibly back as far as primitive man - who may have stumbled across the use of plants and herbs by observing the effect of burning certain twigs, and also by observing the plants that sick animals chose to eat.

The Egyptians were using aromatics almost 5,000 years ago for both medicinal and cosmetic purposes, as well as for embalming their dead. We have learnt from papyrus documents of some of the herbs and plants used, along with the methods they adopted. Although they did not know how to distil the essential oils, they did make pills, powders, ointments and pastes.

The ancient Greeks used the knowledge acquired from the Egyptians to make a few discoveries of their own. For example, they used olive oil to absorb odour from flower petals and herbs, and used perfumed oil for both medicinal and cosmetic purposes. There is also recorded evidence to show that Greek soldiers carried ointment of myrrh for wounds endured through battle.

Word spread and the Arab world began research into plant uses in medicine, with Avicenna, one of the greatest Arab physicians being credited with the discovery of distilling essential oils. It now seems more likely that he perfected, rather than invented, the technique as archaeologists have found primitive drawings that pre-date his lifetime, but he refined the method by adding cooling coils.

The use of plants for healing in the Far East, especially India and China, is recorded in some of the most ancient religious texts, one as far back as 2,000 BC, which contain formulae using benzoin, caraway, clove, ginger, pepper and sandalwood.

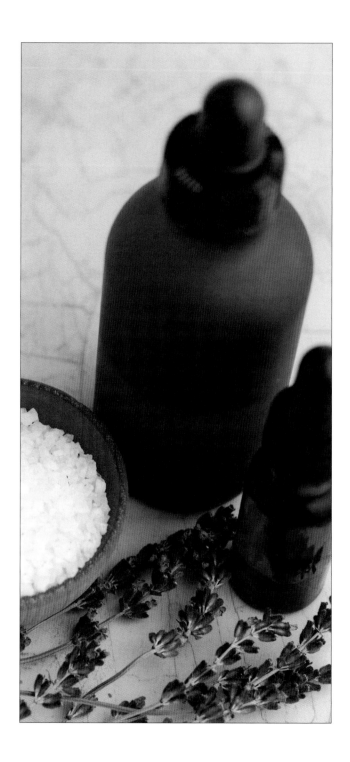

In Europe we know that by the 12th century the 'perfumes of Arabia', or essential oils, were brought back by crusading knights, along with the knowledge of how to distil them. In the 17th century there followed an inclination towards the then new use of chemical substances in medicine, with the use of herbs and plants being seen as outmoded or archaic in comparison to the new pharmaceutical drugs. This also coincided with a spate of witch burning by the religious establishment who were deeply suspicious of village 'wise women' and saw its practice as heresy. Thankfully, attitudes are a little more tolerant today!

During the 1920s in France, Rene Maurice Gattefosse, a chemist in his family's perfume company, became interested in the medicinal aspect of essential oils. He discovered that many of the essential oils were better antiseptics than the chemical ones being added to the products.

He burnt his hand badly in a lab explosion and plunged it into some neat lavender oil; it healed amazingly quickly, with no infection or scarring. He then continued to use essential oils to treat soldiers during World War 1. This led him to develop the use of essential oils in dermatology and to undertake extensive research into their medicinal applications.

In 1941 the British Pharmacy and Medicines Act made the practice of herbal medicine illegal. Then, some 60 years later, the scientific world is reappraising the value of natural remedies: as the limited effectiveness, and unwanted side-effects, of aggressive, synthesised medications are becoming recognised, aromatic essences are back in vogue.

What is aromatherapy?

- Aromatherapy is a holistic therapy, treating both body and mind.

- It is an ancient art that uses essential oil extracts for cosmetic and therapeutic treatments, using odiferous substances obtained from plants and aromatic shrubs.

- Aromatherapy works on many different levels and is unique in its multi-faceted benefits - the aroma has an effect on your mood, application through massage comforts and relaxes you, and the individual properties of the oils will have their own effect on the body

- It is the principle of using carefully selected blends of essential oils to help alleviate various problems such as stress and fatigue. The oils can be massaged into the skin, applied in a compress, inhaled or bathed in.

- It is a natural remedy, derived directly from plants, which encourages individual responsibility for health as essential oils play an increasing part in home treatments for everyday conditions such as headaches, fatigue, stress and aches and pains.

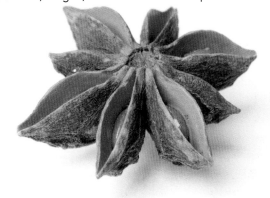

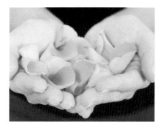

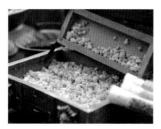

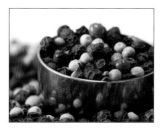

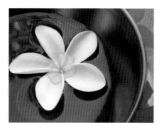

What are Essential Oils?

Essential oils are not actually oils at all but in fact plant hormones extracted in tiny quantities from the blossom, leaves, fruit, seeds, stems, balsam, resin, bark, wood and root of the various plants. They differ from other oils as, due to their watery substance, they do not leave oily marks. They are highly volatile, and evaporate quickly on contact with air, and are lighter than water. They are generally colourless, highly flammable, odiferous and soluble in oil and alcohol.

They have many individual and varied benefits - some are antibacterial, antifungal, antiseptic, anti-inflammatory, or a combination of all! This makes them particularly useful and helps to build up immunity and protect us against bacteria and viruses, along with helping us combat the negative affects of the fast pace of 21st-century life. Essential oils do all of this without damaging the body tissues, and can be readily employed by many different people in a variety of ways, rather than being limited to the hands of the health professional.

Quality Issues

Many factors can influence the quality of essential oils. The same plants grown in different regions, under different conditions and harvested in different ways can produce essential oils of widely diverse characteristics. Just as with wines, there are good and bad years.

The distillation in Europe is centred in Grasse in the South of France – this is the most important centre for the distillation of essential oils. For ingredients, herbs generally tend to be grown in more temperate climates, whilst the majority of spices originate in tropical countries.

- Quality of the soil - soils devoid of nutrients and contaminated by chemical pesticides and herbicides will not cultivate as pure a quality oil as those of organic and nutrient-rich soils

- Altitude at which the plants are grown - this affects the purity of the air as well as the humidity

- Country of origin - this is reflected in the climate of a given country, and the degree of pollutants existing in that country

- Climate conditions - humid climates best suit herbs whereas spices would not flourish under such inclement weather conditions

- Time of year the plant is harvested - rather like food, if harvested too early or too late the quality of the plant is compromised

- Time of day the crop is harvested - various flowers are best picked before dawn, whereas some herbs need harvesting mid-afternoon or at dusk

- How the crop is stored prior to extraction - wooden crates and Hessian sacks will not alter the quality of the essential oil, in comparison to metal or plastic containers, which will most certainly compromise the quality of the oil

- Method of distillation - steam distillation offers the least amount of contamination and produces the purest quality of oil

All of these factors greatly affect the price of the essential oil, which is why there is such a variance on the high street, and with skincare companies who retail oils or products rich in essential oils. The price of oil is also subject to the amount of raw material required to produce a small amount of essence.

For example, we have all experienced the profusion of essential oil in an orange peel: it actually squirts out when we peel it and fills the air with its characteristic aroma. But not all plants contain essential oils in such profusion.

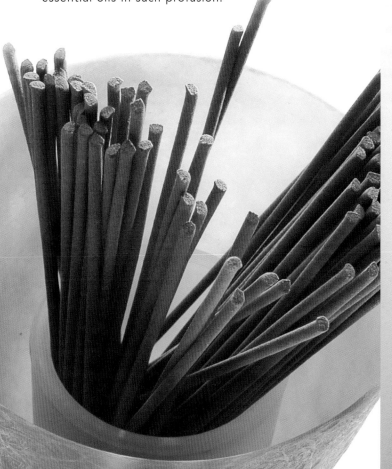

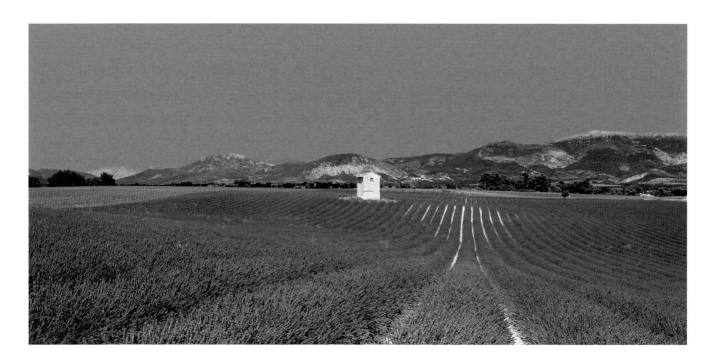

Methods of Extraction

Essential oils are very difficult to extract from petals, leaves, roots and fruits, and different methods are used in doing so, depending on the type of plant material in which the oil is found. Some plant materials, especially flowers, are subject to deterioration and should be processed as soon as possible after harvesting. Others, including seeds and roots, are either stored or transported for extraction to Europe or America. Essential oils have individual fragrances and are composed of complex chemical constituents and elements including alcohols, esters, hydrocarbons, aldehydes, ketones, phenols, terpene alcohols and acids. This means that modern chemists are able to synthesise essential oils with almost 100% accuracy, and, because of the high cost of extracting pure essential oils from some plants, many synthetic oils are produced, making it difficult for all but an expert to tell the difference.

There are two main methods of extraction, expression or pressure, as is the case with most citrus oils. Extraction by steam, water or dry distillation is also used.

Dry steam distillation

Very similar to steam distillation except that the plant material is not placed in water but steam is passed through instead.

Expression

This method is used mainly to extract essential oils from citrus fruits. The peel is scratched or crushed between rollers and the oil can then be separated from the pith by spinning the mixed pulp in a centrifuging machine.

Solvent extraction

Various chemicals are used as solvents, which boil at a low heat until completely evaporated. This produces a solid mass, called a concrete, which can be further treated with alcohol to produce an absolute. This is a highly concentrated form of essential oil.

Maceration

This is a method sometimes used with flowers that lose their fragrance almost immediately after picking. The flowers are dipped into hot fat, which absorbs the essential oils from the plant. As with enfleurage (see below), alcohol then separates the oils from the fat.

Hydro diffusion

Similar to steam distillation except that the steam enters at the top of the still, above the plant material. This is more suited to wood and fibrous material.

Enfleurage

This process involves cold fat and is a labour-intensive method used for flowers that continue to generate essential oils after they have been harvested, for example jasmine. A sheet of glass, mounted into a wooden frame, is spread with a thin layer of pure, odourless fat. A layer of flowers is sprinkled onto the fat. After 24-30 hours the flowers have given up their essential oils to the fat. The used flowers are discarded and fresh ones added. This process is repeated several times, sometimes over a long period, until the fat is saturated with essential oils. Known as pomade, this is washed in alcohol and the essential oils pass into the alcohol.

The alcohol is then evaporated leaving pure essential oils.

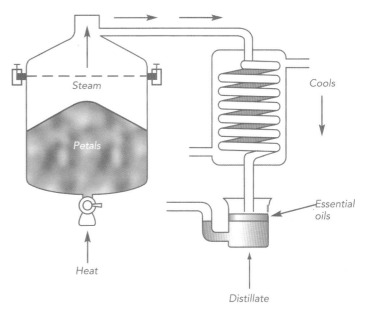

Steam distillation

By far the oldest and most widely used method of extraction is by steam distillation. The plant material is placed in a container along with a volume of water. It is heated to boiling point and the mixture evaporates. In the steam are molecules of essential oil, which have been released from the plant by the heating process.

The steam and the essential oil molecules rise and enter a downward running coiled pipe. The coiled pipe is cooled by refrigerated water passing around it, which cools the steam and returns it to the liquid. This liquid contains small amounts of the essential oil mixed with a watery residue called distillate. These separate, making it easy to siphon the essential oil off the top.

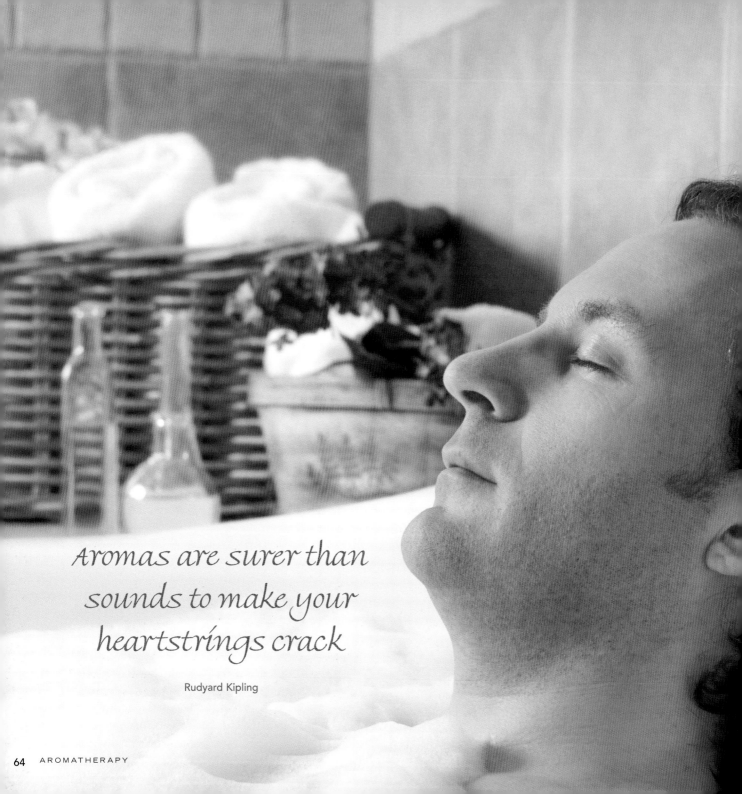

Aromas are surer than sounds to make your heartstrings crack

Rudyard Kipling

How Do Essential Oils Work?

There are three main ways in which essential oils can have an effect on the body:

- Inhalation

- Absorption through the skin

- Ingestion (administered by a medical practitioner only)

In order to gain an understanding of the way essential oils work, it is probably helpful to take an overall view of each of the body's systems.

The skin
Essential oils enter the skin in several ways. They enter through hair follicles or sweat glands and are then absorbed into the blood vessels through the capillary network. The oils can pass efficiently through tissue because their molecular structure is small enough to penetrate fatty layers and travel through interstitial fluid. Some essential oils with smaller molecular structures may also travel directly through the cell.

Massage
Application to the skin can be in a number of ways - massage, bathing and compress being the most pleasurable. With massage, always try to use the same essential oil in an aromatic burner to achieve optimum therapeutic benefits. This is because there is no blood supply to the deep brain and so body massage will therefore have limited use, whereas burning oils will have an immediate effect on the mind and emotional health of your client.

Compress
Hot and cold compresses can be used with appropriate oils for injuries, aches and pains, severe tension, headaches, abscesses and indigestion. The compress should be slightly wet and not dripping with water, and needs to be applied over the affected area and left on for 10-15 minutes.

A hot compress is good for backache, severe tension, earache, arthritic or rheumatic pain. A cold compress helps to treat headache, migraine, bruises, sprains and inflammation (hot swellings).

Bathing
This is the easiest and most pleasurable way of using essential oils for therapeutic benefit. Remember to always add the oils to the bath once it is full: the oils are volatile and will lose much of their therapeutic value under running water.

A warm bath has a calming and soothing effect on both the body and mind, a hot bath is stimulating and valuable for encouraging elimination of wastes and detoxification, and a cool bath has a more revitalising and energising effect.

Inhalation
This is our forgotten sense in many ways. Our sense of smell is one of the most widely misunderstood and neglected functions of the human body. This is ironic when we consider that for early man our sense of smell was essential to survival.

If we are to understand how essential oils can affect our mind and emotions, we need to understand the physical mechanisms involved. Our sense of smell is the direct link between our brain and the environment we are in. Only 3 inches separate the olfactory receptor sites (in the nose) and the brain; the nerve fibres of the olfactory system run directly to the limbic area of the brain (the 'old' or 'smell' brain). It is thought to have developed more than 70 million years ago and is why, through scent, we have a direct link to our distant past.

The olfactory cells are the only nerve cells that regenerate, and are the only body system to bypass the blood-brain barrier. This is extremely important therapeutically and shows how we can influence moods and emotions so quickly and effectively through the inhalation of essential oils. Consider the following comparison as evidence of how quickly inhalation influences the body systems: cyanide kills in 2-3 minutes when ingested but only 10 seconds if inhaled.

Use essential oils in a vaporiser, diffuser, light bulb ring (not directly on the bulb as it will cause it to explode), steam inhalation and scented in fabrics or burning logs.

Ingestion
Due to the concentrated nature of essential oils, it is not recommended that clients ingest oils unless prescribed by a medically qualified practitioner.

Amazingly, just 5ml of eucalyptus oil is enough to kill a fully grown man.

Essential Oils for the Skin

There are many essential oils that are valuable for the skincare therapist when working to achieve effective results for clients. Using oils such as sandalwood, geranium, palmarosa, myrrh, frankincense and bergamot will all be beneficial for a wide range of skincare needs. Yet, there are five essential oils that produce consistently fabulous results for skincare concerns and so are especially valuable. This is partly due to their mildness and compatibility to the skin but also because they enjoy powerful medicinal properties.

~ Rose ~

Rosa Damascena - country of origin is Bulgaria; taken from the flower

It is one of the most useful skincare oils because, apart from its rich, feminine scent, it has good wound-healing properties, which help in the daily process of skin repair. Rose is especially valuable for use as a solution for broken capillaries, or thread veins, due to its astringent effect on the capillaries, which helps to diminish the redness.

For general skincare, rose is suited to:

- All types of complexion

- Broken capillaries

- Wrinkles

- Conjunctivitis

- Dry skin

- Eczema

- Herpes

- Maturing and sensitised skin

For general factors that may be affecting the skin, rose helps relieve:

- Depression

- Insomnia

- Nervous tension

- Headaches

- Stress-related conditions

- Liver function

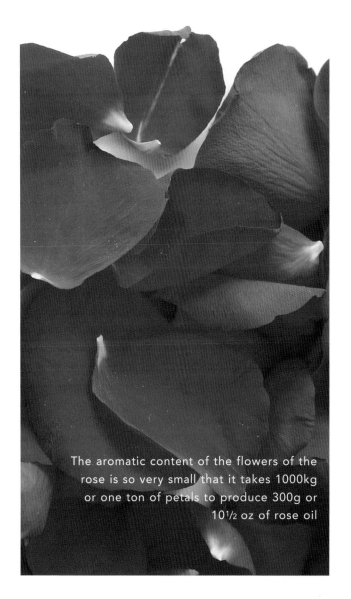

The aromatic content of the flowers of the rose is so very small that it takes 1000kg or one ton of petals to produce 300g or 10½ oz of rose oil

~ Neroli ~

Citrus Aurantium - country of origin China; from flowers of the orange blossom

This oil has powerful bactericidal and antiseptic agents with excellent cytophylactic properties, encouraging the formation of new skin cells. Similar to rose and lavender, they have the most hauntingly beautiful scent, which is uplifting, fresh and citrus-like. It can safely be used in pregnancy and can be blended with mandarin to prevent stretch marks.

For general skincare, neroli is suited to:

- Scars

- Stretch marks

- Thread veins

- Maturing and sensitised skin

- Toning the complexion

- Wrinkles

For general factors that may be affecting the skin, neroli helps relieve:

- Anxiety

- Grief and emotional trauma

- Depression

- Nervous tension

- Stress-related conditions

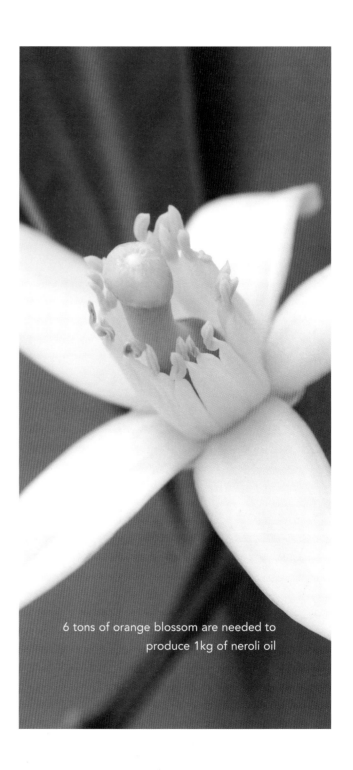

6 tons of orange blossom are needed to produce 1kg of neroli oil

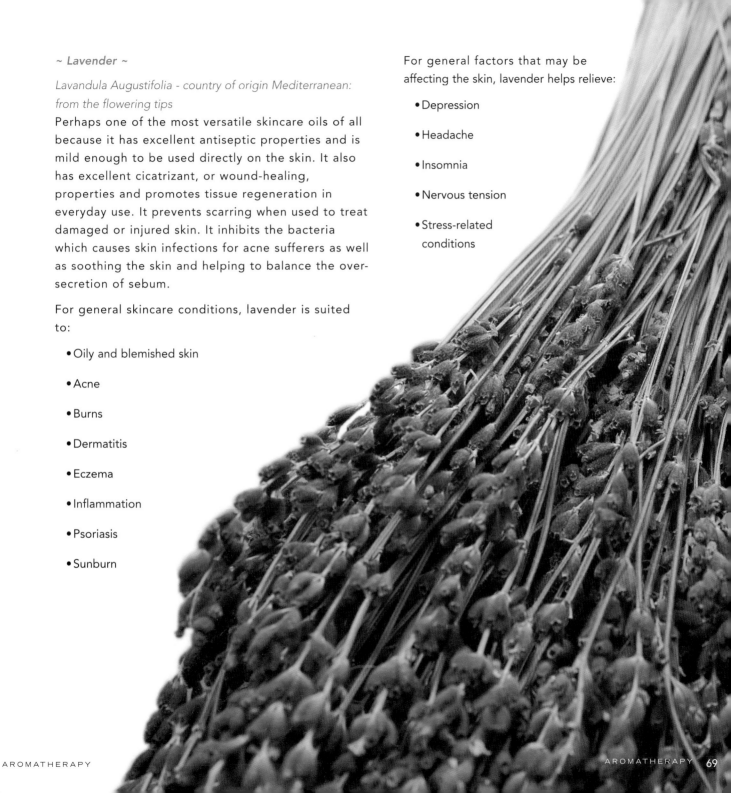

~ Lavender ~

Lavandula Augustifolia - country of origin Mediterranean:
from the flowering tips

Perhaps one of the most versatile skincare oils of all because it has excellent antiseptic properties and is mild enough to be used directly on the skin. It also has excellent cicatrizant, or wound-healing, properties and promotes tissue regeneration in everyday use. It prevents scarring when used to treat damaged or injured skin. It inhibits the bacteria which causes skin infections for acne sufferers as well as soothing the skin and helping to balance the over-secretion of sebum.

For general skincare conditions, lavender is suited to:

- Oily and blemished skin

- Acne

- Burns

- Dermatitis

- Eczema

- Inflammation

- Psoriasis

- Sunburn

For general factors that may be affecting the skin, lavender helps relieve:

- Depression

- Headache

- Insomnia

- Nervous tension

- Stress-related conditions

~ Tea tree ~

Melaleuca Alternifolia - country of origin Australia: from the leaves and twigs

A valuable skincare oil because, apart from patchouli, it is the only essential oil that has excellent antiseptic, fungicidal, and antiviral properties, yet is still mild on the skin. Particularly good for infected skin conditions, especially for fungal infections. This oil can be used to strengthen the immune system prior to surgery and can also be helpful afterwards to reduce post-operative shock.

For general skincare conditions, tea tree is suited to:

- Cold sores
- Acne
- Herpes
- Oily skin
- Spots
- Rashes

For general factors that may be affecting the skin, tea tree:

- Stimulates the immune system
- Help scars to heal

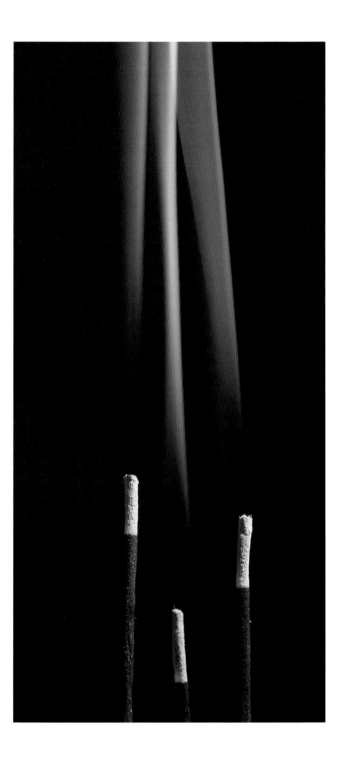

~ Chamomile ~

Matricaria Recutica - country of origin Europe; from the flower

Chamomile is a well-known soothing remedy, and because of its sedative and relaxant properties it is particularly good for all types of skin complaints that have a nervous or stress-related element. The properties of chamomile and lavender often overlap so it may be useful to remember that as an analgesic, chamomile is better for dull aches and pains, while lavender may be better for sharp, piercing pain and inflammation.

For general skincare conditions, chamomile is suited to:

- Acne

- Boils

- Burns

- Cuts

- Dermatitis

- Eczema

- Inflammation and allergies

- Sensitised skin

For general factors that may be affecting the skin, chamomile helps relieve:

- Insomnia

- Headaches and migraine

- Nervous tension

- Stress-related complaints

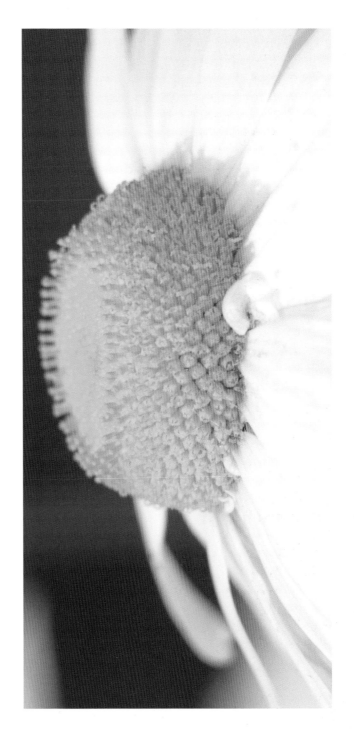

A person's foot is half of their adult size by the age of one.

REFLEXOLOGY

This chapter presents an introduction to reflexology, offers an understanding of what type of condition is helped by the treatment and summarises the benefits. It is not designed to equip you to practise as a reflexologist, but should go some way toward informing your thinking when working with clients.

What Exactly is Reflexology?

This is likely to be the most commonly asked question when you're advising a client to seek the professional help of a reflexologist.

It is a form of natural, holistic therapy based on the discovery that certain points on the hands and feet correspond to systems, organs and structures in the entire body. It can be described as a specialised form of massage of the hands and feet, but most commonly the feet.

It is, however, far more than simply massage - special pressure techniques are used to detect and correct congestion or 'imbalances' in the body that may be causing ill-health. It is a highly relaxing yet deeply stimulating treatment using the principles of therapeutic human touch and interaction to work with the body's natural healing systems.

The Earliest Indication of Foot Therapy

There is evidence that reflexology has its roots in the practices of the healers of ancient Egypt, Greece, Rome and China. The oldest evidence documenting a treatment given to the feet is from an Egyptian papyrus from 2,300 BC, which shows physicians working on the feet and hands of two patients. There is also evidence to suggest

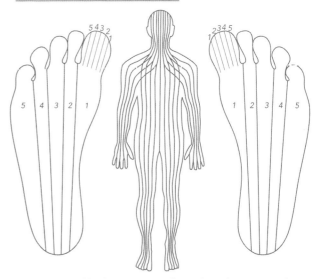

> *The Ten Energy Zones of the Body*

> *In Dr Fitzgerald's theory, energy flows through ten vertical zones that run from the feet to the head, and also down each arm to the hands.*
> *Pressure on a reflex point in the appropriate zone area on the foot can treat organs, glands, bones and muscles within that zone.*

reflexology was used for healing amongst the native peoples of both North and South America.

From Ayurvedic medicine, we know that a form of pressure technique on the feet is used as part of their system of 'Marma' points. Similarly, Chinese acupressure and acupuncture use many points located on the feet. The principle of all of these cultures was to take a comprehensive view of the person and their disease, rather than the traditional Western view of seeing them as totally separate.

What is accepted is that no one culture can claim authorship of this ancient therapy: therapeutic touch of the feet has been in existence in many cultures of the ancient world.

Reflexology as we know it today has evolved largely from the work of two Americans from the early 20th century, Dr William Fitzgerald and Eunice Ingham (the latter was an American physiotherapist). It was Fitzgerald who first proposed the theory that the body is divided into ten equal zones that extend the length of the body, and that stimulating the foot in one zone affects the other parts of the body in the same zone.

It was Eunice Ingham who developed the body chart, which, she claimed, shows how the entire body is reflected in the soles and sides of both feet. One of her students, Doreen Bayley, introduced reflexology to the UK in the 1960s and popularity has since soared, not only in the UK but also in Australia and New Zealand.

Not a Diagnostic Tool

Although reflexology has a hugely beneficial effect on the health, it can not be used to diagnose disease such as cancer or heart disease, for example, or to treat other medical conditions.

Reflexologists are not licensed medical practitioners but are trained to assess imbalances in the whole person and work with their natural body systems to help restore balance. Areas of imbalance detected by the practitioner are not always accompanied by symptoms of disease. An imbalance may confirm the existence of an old illness or site of disease, or it may be caused by the new shoes the client is wearing!

Commonsense must prevail at all times.

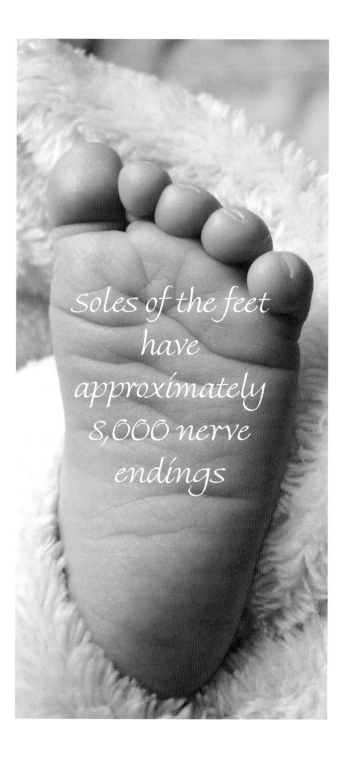

soles of the feet have approximately 8,000 nerve endings

Using Therapeutic Touch

As the feet are being worked on by the reflexologist, imbalances that may exist in the body reflexes can be detected. This can be experienced by the client in the form of tenderness, tingling, sensitivity or, occasionally, acute pain when pressure is applied to a particular point or reflex. These sensations may be accompanied by the therapist sensing changes in the temperature of that area of the foot, a bubble-like popping feeling, or grittiness, sometimes referred to as crystals.

Reflexology helps reconnect and restore the balance between our mind, body and inner emotions. As specialists with a holistic approach, we understand that, like all toxins, negativity accumulates in the most unused and slumbering parts of the body, and negative thoughts and behaviours are no different - they gravitate where the consciousness does not reach.

When a reflexologist works with clarity and unconditional reflection, it can help a client relate some of the sensations to experiences, feelings and mental attitudes that may be contributing to the imbalance. I find it deeply rewarding when clients experience what I describe as a silent 'Aha' moment. This signifies that the client is beginning to take responsibility for the changes they need to make.

Case Study

I worked for some time with a company CEO who was 'sent by his fiancée' and so was deeply cynical about the possible benefits of my 'rubbing his feet'. For months he poked fun, challenged and refused to accept that reflexology was making any difference to his stress levels and mood swings (although curiously he did return each week!)

To begin with he talked throughout most of the treatment, with me acting as a 'mirror' to his thoughts and feelings. He then began to sleep serenely through many more sessions whilst I continued to work on any imbalances, about which he teased me, saying that I waited until he fell asleep and then sat and read a magazine!

The change in his attitude and manner was so subtle but evident nevertheless. The final joy was when the 'foot and mouth woman' (my pet name apparently) was happy to accept an invitation to his forthcoming wedding - his fiancée had finally agreed to marry this 'grumpy git'. To this day he is unable to understand how massaging the feet can have such a profound effect on all areas of his life.
It just does; lets leave it at that.

What conditions can be helped?

- Digestive problems such as constipation and IBS

- Menstrual irregularities

- Stress and stress-related disorders such as anxiety and insomnia

- High blood pressure

- Pain relief

- Inflammatory skin conditions

- Chronic conditions in older people, and children; dementia in older people, or colic in children

- Back pain

- Asthma

- Psoriasis and eczema

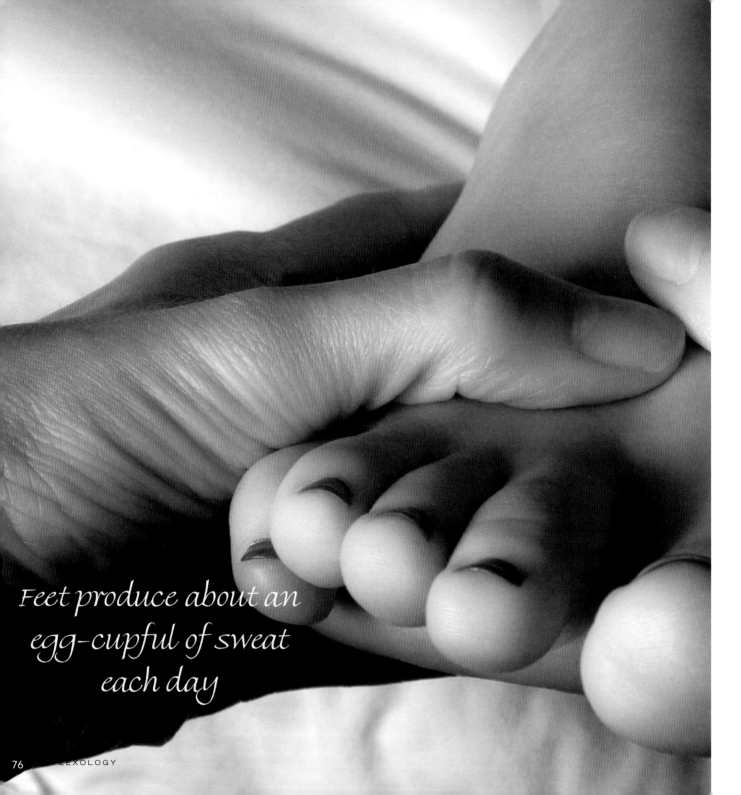

Feet produce about an egg-cupful of sweat each day

Some Common Questions

How long does the treatment last?

Generally between 45 and 60 minutes.

How many sessions will I need?

Depending on the severity of the problem, several weekly sessions may be advised. Many people have regular treatments to maintain well-being.

Will it hurt or be uncomfortable?

A reflex point may be tender if there is an imbalance, but this eases in the hands of a professional practitioner who will adjust the pressure to suit your sensitivity. Ticklish feet should also not be a problem.

What are the after-effects?

Sometimes people have what is described as a healing crisis - a rash, runny nose, urge to urinate or a cough. This is the body's natural healing process to remove the toxins stirred up by the treatment.

Main benefits

- Reduces stress and induces deep relaxation

- Improves circulation

- Cleanses the body of toxins and impurities

- Balances the whole body system

- Revitalises energy

- Is great for preventative health care

- Creates a feeling of well-being

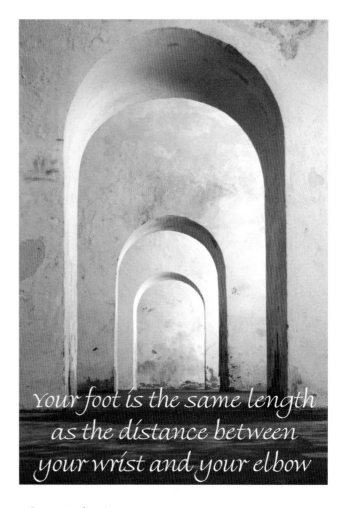

Your foot is the same length as the distance between your wrist and your elbow

Contra-indications

- First trimester (three months) of pregnancy

- Thyroid problems, diabetes or long-term health problems - treatment only with GP consent

- Someone taking a course of homeopathic medicine

- Long-term use of medication - could potentially upset the action of the dose due to stimulation and increased blood flow

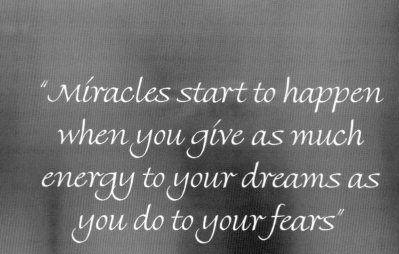

"Miracles start to happen when you give as much energy to your dreams as you do to your fears"

Richard Wilkins

ACUPRESSURE

The objective of this chapter is to give you an understanding of acupressure and the pressure points that are helpful for a skincare therapist. It also demonstrates the benefits of teaching some basic pressure points to your clients. There are easy steps that can be shown to your clients to help relieve stress-related problems, both physical and emotional. This allows them to actively participate in their own healing - something they will love you for.

As with previous chapters, the aim is to inform and familiarise. It is well worth the additional reading to understand more fully the application of this wonderful and highly effective practice. Alternatively, get to know a practitioner in your area to whom you can confidently refer clients when the need arises; their loyalty to you will return ten-fold!

Acupressure can be used to treat many different health problems, for example allergies, muscular and skeletal problems, arthritis, asthma and breathing difficulties, cramps, spasms, earache, impotency and labour pains. However, we are going to concentrate on the acupressure points related to the skin, and areas that commonly affect the condition of the skin.

What is Acupressure?

The origins of acupressure are as ancient as the instinctive impulse to hold your head or temples when you have a headache. Everyone at one time or another has used their hands spontaneously to hold or rub tense and painful places of the body.

Acupressure is an ancient healing art that uses fingers to press key points on the surface of the skin to stimulate the body's natural healing abilities. When these points are pressed, they release muscular tension and promote increased circulation of the blood and lymphatic systems.

As with reflexology and aromatherapy, acupressure was conceived in Asian cultures using the knowledge and understanding of energy pathways in the body. The Chinese call this chi and the Japanese call it ki.

Stimulating these points with pressure, needles or heat triggers releases endorphins and neurochemicals that relieve pain. As a result, pain is blocked and the flow of blood and oxygen to the affected area is increased. This causes the muscles to relax and promotes healing. Because acupressure inhibits the pain signals sent to the brain, it has been described as closing the 'gates' of the pain-signalling system, preventing the painful sensations from passing through the spinal cord to the brain.

Besides relieving pain, acupressure can help rebalance the body by easing tensions and stresses (both of which inhibit the immune system) that keep it from functioning smoothly. Tension tends to concentrate around acupressure points. When a muscle is chronically tense or in spasm, the muscle fibres contract due to the production of lactic acid caused by fatigue, trauma, stress, chemical imbalances or poor circulation. For example, as detailed in the chapter on stress, the breathing of a stressed person may become shallow; certain acupressure points can relieve chest tension, enabling the stressed client to breathe deeply once more.

As a point is pressed, the muscle tension yields to the finger pressure, enabling the fibres to elongate and relax, the blood to flow freely, and toxins to be released and eliminated. Increased blood and lymph circulation then brings fresh oxygen and other nutrients to the affected area. When the blood circulates properly, we achieve a greater sense of harmony, health and well-being. This is never more evident than with the complexion: increased blood and lymphatic circulation helps to rejuvenate and firm the skin, along with improving the skin's condition and muscle tone. The accompanying relaxation of the facial muscles is one of the most effective, drug-free anti-ageing products available!

Acupressure is a natural way to balance the body and maintain good health. The healing touch of this ancient system reduces tension, increases circulation and enables the body to enter a state of deep relaxation. By relieving stress, acupressure strengthens resistance to disease and promotes a feeling of well-being.

Acupuncture and acupressure use the same points but acupuncture employs needles, whilst acupressure uses the gentle pressure of the hands (and sometimes the feet!) For the holistic therapist, acupressure will be the most effective method for treatment as it is easily taught to clients, and can treat tension-related ailments by using the power and sensitivity of the hands. You can, with a little imagination, teach clients to practise acupressure anywhere and at anytime.

Acupressure Massage Techniques

For the purposes of facial acupressure, we will concentrate on the massage techniques relevant to this area. There are several other techniques that are used on the body; please refer to the reading list if you would like to discover more about these.

Firm pressure - this is the primary technique.

- For the face, use fingers and thumbs to apply a steady, fixed pressure.

- Gently hold each point for a minute or more.

- Pressing with an intermittent, fast beat is stimulating; a slower pressure creates a deeply relaxing effect.

- To relax an area or to ease pain, apply pressure gradually and hold for longer periods - one minute of steady pressure calms and relaxes the nervous system, promoting greater healing.

- To stimulate an area, apply pressure for only 4 or 5 seconds at a time.

Slow motion kneading - for working across the neck and shoulders to relieve tension and general stiffness.

- Use the thumbs and fingers along with the heel of the hands to squeeze large muscles, such as across the trapezius and deltoids.

- Use a squeezing and lifting motion, or try kneading (like a mass of bread dough). To reduce fatigue, lean the weight of your upper body into this movement rather than using your hands to apply pressure. It should be a squeeze rather than a nip, so ensure you use fingers, thumbs and hands.

Quick tapping - for stimulating non-fleshy areas.

- Use fingertips or pads of fingers in a rapid but light movement.

- Improves the functioning of the nerves.

- Stimulates muscle tone.

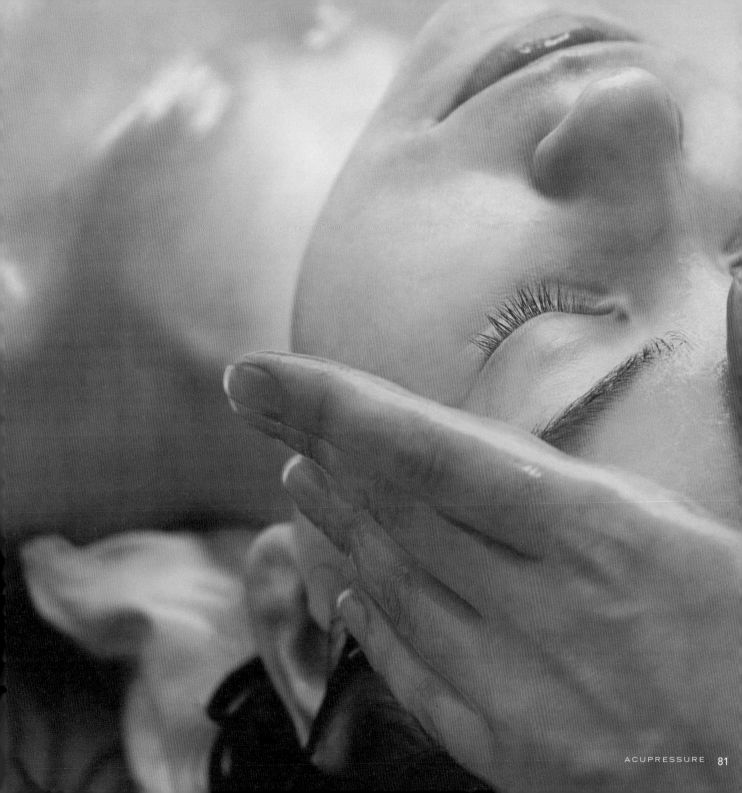

- Always apply finger pressure in a slow, rhythmic style to enable the different layers of tissue to respond.

- The middle finger is the longest and strongest finger and is best suited to applying pressure; the thumb is also strong but not sensitive enough for working on the face.

- Apply a slow, firm pressure at a 90° angle. If the skin is pulled in any way, the angle is wrong.

- Apply and release the pressure applied gradually. This allows the tissues to respond and repair. End each pressure with about 20 seconds of light touch.

- The better your concentration when working on an area, the more effective the treatment will be.

- Never press any area in an abrupt, forceful or jarring way as this is not only deeply unpleasant but can also cause pain and possible bruising.

- Keep your fingernails trimmed fairly short to avoid scratching, possible discomfort or, even worse, injury to the client's skin.

- For optimal results, encourage clients to practise the routine daily, although 2 to 3 times a week can still be effective.

- Limit the sessions to an hour at the most, but do not work on a single area for more than 15 minutes. For example: 15 minutes on the face, 15 minutes on the neck and 15 minutes on the shoulders.

- Sometimes you will get 'referred pain'. This is pain experienced somewhere other than the point you are working on, and indicates that the areas are connected. Press points in these areas as well to release blockages.

- After repeated sessions, you will begin to feel a pulse at each point. This is a good sign and means the circulation has increased.

- If your hand becomes fatigued, withdraw the pressure, gently shake out your hand, take some deep breathes and then resume.

Deep Breathing

Without correct breathing, true relaxation is impossible and peace of mind is hard to achieve. Poor breathing affects the body in other ways, sapping energy, undermining the immune system, making the body prone to illness and making us irritable.

Learning to breathe naturally has two immediate benefits that are much in demand in the modern world. It secretly removes fatigue and refreshes the mind and body. Natural breathing can transform weary nerves into a state of relaxation in a very short time and, like a magic wand, can melt away feelings of exhaustion and replace them with vitality and oomph!

Deep breathing is one of the most intensely effective tools for a therapist to use with a highly stressed or anxious client. It is 'best practice' to start any treatment with deep breathing exercises, but particularly when working on energy lines or meridians during acupressure or reflexology treatments. Deep breathing also helps the acupressure points release any pain or tension and encourages the healing energy to flow throughout the body.

~ How to breathe ~

- Either lie on the floor or sit upright in a chair.

- Place each hand lightly on the rib cage, parallel with the 'floating' or bottom ribs.

- Concentrate on what is happening with the chest.

- Start with a long, slow exhalation (breath out). Concentrate on feeling the bottom ribs: if they are still, press them gently inward.

- Draw inhaled air from the nose not the mouth. Feel the ribs move outward.

- On the breath in, the abdominal muscles should tense slightly.

- On the breath out, they should relax.

- Expel air through the nose not the mouth.

- Repeat for up to 5 minutes.

- Relax before getting up again.

For many people, trying to breathe in this way is so difficult it makes them realise just how bad their breathing has become. Persevere; the benefits are very worth it.

The healing benefits of acupressure involve both the relaxation of the body and its positive effects on the mind. As tension is released we not only feel great physically, but we feel better emotionally and mentally. When the body relaxes the mind relaxes as well, creating a deeper state of awareness or consciousness. This expanded awareness leads to mental clarity and a healthier physical and emotional being, melting away the division between mind and body.

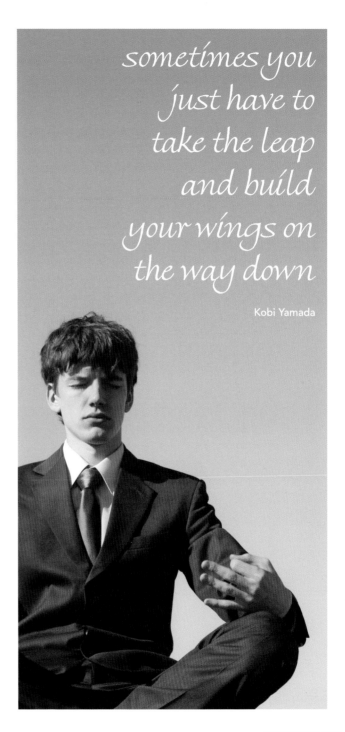

sometimes you just have to take the leap and build your wings on the way down

Kobi Yamada

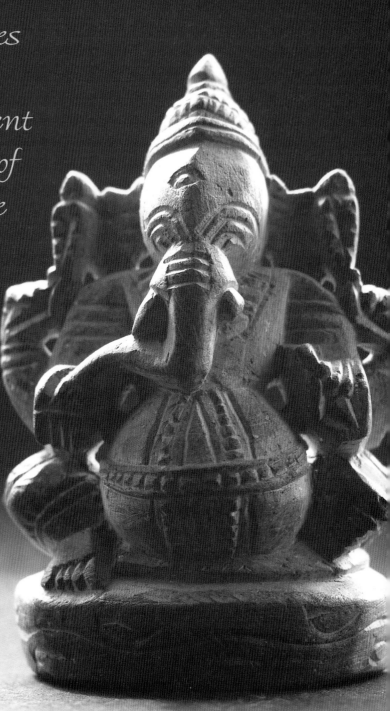

"What we are today comes from our thoughts of yesterday, and our present thoughts build our life of tomorrow: our life is the creation of our mind"

Buddha

AYURVEDA

The purpose of this chapter is to explain the ancient, holistic system of medicine of Ayurveda in simple terms to those who may have heard of it but know very little about it and would like to learn more. There are those in the UK who have described this ancient healing system as 'the sleeping giant of complementary medicine'.

The objective is to offer an insight into this sophisticated and comprehensive health system, and hopefully support the ambitions of the skincare detective by offering a shorthand technique towards uncovering the unspoken aspects of a client's personality and uniqueness.

What is Ayurveda?

Ayurveda (pronounced eye-yer-vay-duh) is from the ancient Indian language, Sanskrit, and literally means 'Knowledge or Wisdom of Life'. Ayur means life and ved means knowledge. Inherent in Ayurvedic principles is the concept that we are capable of taking charge of our own life and healing. The purpose of Ayurvedic medicine is to avoid serious illness by having a thorough understanding of how we become ill. It has a strong interest in prevention. But when illness does strike, Ayurveda has a wide range of treatments that help the body to heal itself.

All Ayurvedic treatments are natural, herb-based remedies - a contrast to allopathic medicine's drugs, which are concocted in test tubes and subject to the whims of fashionable thought from the various drugs companies. Ayurveda's treatments are ancient, have stood the test of time and have no harmful side-effects.

This traditional healing system of the Indian subcontinent covers all aspects of health, encouraging physical, mental, emotional and spiritual well-being. It is the oldest and most complete medical system in the world, dating back to 3000 BC and has similarities with Traditional Chinese Medicine (TCM). Unlike orthodox medicine, it is not based on the frequently changing findings of specific research projects, but rather on permanent, wise, eternal principles of living.

Ayurveda may come from ancient texts, but the principles and approaches are just as applicable today in our fast-paced, high-pressure society as they were when originally recorded in India. In fact, along with Buddhism, it is the fastest growing belief system in the West. It complements orthodox Western medicine and, because it understands how and why we become ill, it can offer effective treatment for many conditions for which conventional medicine has not found a cure.

In the same way that aromatherapy was once seen as outmoded or archaic, the principal systems of Ayurvedic medicine were once in danger of being replaced altogether by Western medicine. Thankfully, in 1980 the National Congress of India decided that Ayurveda should enjoy equal status with Western medicine and so funded many new Ayurvedic institutions. It, too, has enjoyed something of a renaissance since the 1980s.

Fundamental Elements

Ayurveda teaches us that those highly complex organisms we call human beings are made up of a mixture of matter and anti-matter, and that it is the constant interaction between those two which determines the state of our physical and mental health.

Ayurveda's most powerful belief is that nothing functions in isolation and that where there is imbalance the result is illness and disorder.

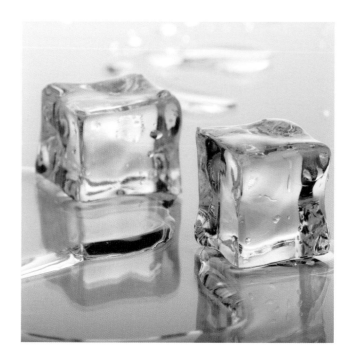

The concepts of life force or energy and balance within the body are as important in Ayurvedic as in Chinese medicine. In Ayurvedic medicine, the life force is prana, similar to the Chinese chi (pronounced chee). As in Chinese medicine, the functioning of the body is controlled by immaterial forces, linked to physical substances.

The human is viewed as a microcosm of the universe, and both the body and the universe can be seen partly in terms of the five elements. In Ayurveda these are space or Ether and Air, Fire, Water and Earth, and the human body is composed of a combination of them. These also correspond with the five cognitive senses of hearing, touch, sight, taste, smell. These five elements may be present in all matter.

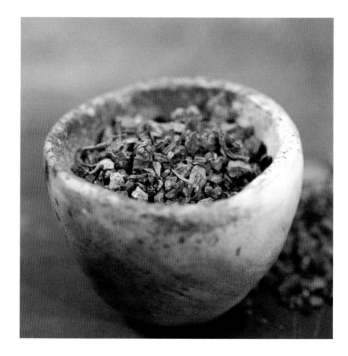

Water is necessary to taste (a dry tongue can not distinguish flavours) and Earth is connected with the sense of smell - the nose relates to the excretory organs, which is why people with constipation often have bad breath and a diminished sense of smell. As always with Ayurveda, everything ties up with everything else. There is harmony and synchronicity, and it is disharmony that creates illness. Ayurvedic treatment aims to recreate harmony as far as possible.

Three principal bio-energies, known as doshas, exist in all things and are composed of different combinations of the five elements. These are rather similar to the Western idea of three basic body types: ectomorph, lean and delicate; mesomorph, compact and muscular; endomorph, stocky. But most of us are a combination of two (or sometimes all three) types, with one predominant.

The doshas are three constantly fluctuating energy qualities that define all things on earth. Each is made up of a combination of two of the five great elements of Ayurveda: Vata is formed from air and ether, Pitta from fire and water, and Kapha from water and earth.

Each individual has a unique combination of doshas, known as prakriti, which is determined by the doshas of their parents at the time of conception. Physiological strengths and weaknesses, intellectual capacity and personality are governed by one or, in some people, two dominant doshas.

Ayurvedic practitioners believe that good health depends on pacifying excesses in the doshas and keeping fluctuations to a minimum. Each dosha has a seat in the body that is able to absorb and eliminate small excesses, but disease can result if the seat cannot cope with larger imbalances.

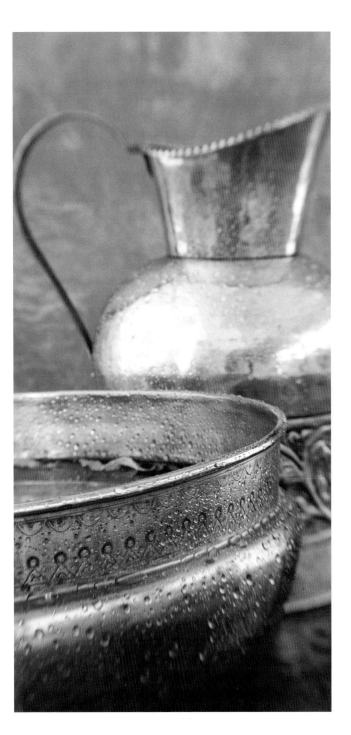

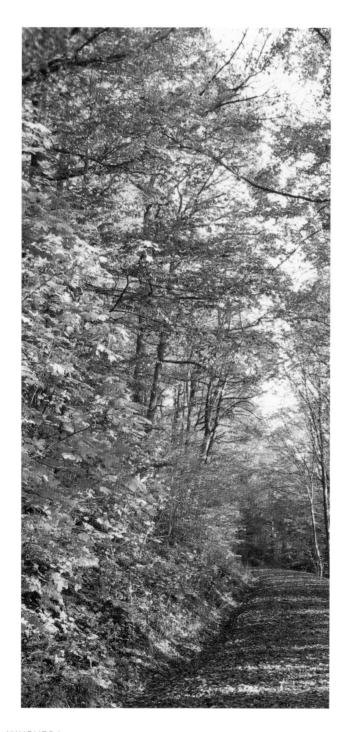

Vata

This is the lightest of the doshas, portrayed by the colour blue. It is linked to the wind, the force that controls movement and the functioning of the nervous system.

- Vata types are either tall or short and of slight build.

- They are creative, with quick, nervous movements but tend to waste energy through restlessness.

- The dominant element is air, then ether.

- The seat of the Vata is the colon.

- A shared quality with Kapha is coldness.

- Tastes that increase Vata are pungent, bitter, astringent. Vata types should avoid raw foods.

- Tastes that pacify Vata are sweet, sour, salty, moist, warming foods such as casseroles and cooked root vegetables.

- The Vata season is autumn and early winter.

- Massage pressure should be light and movement needs to be slow and deliberate.

Characteristics of Vata include:

- A variable appetite

- Little perspiration

- Frequent but sparse urine, hard, dark stools and tendency to constipation

- Highly original and creative mind

- Poor to average memory

- Indecisive

- Rapid speech

- Wastefulness with money

- Nervousness and shyness

- Tendency to anxiety and depression

- High sex drive (or none at all)

- Love of travel

- High mobility

- Dislike of cold weather and strong winds

Health problems associated with Vata include:

- Heart problems

- Disorders of the nervous system

- Anxiety and tension

- Hypertension

- Depression

- Migraine

- IBS

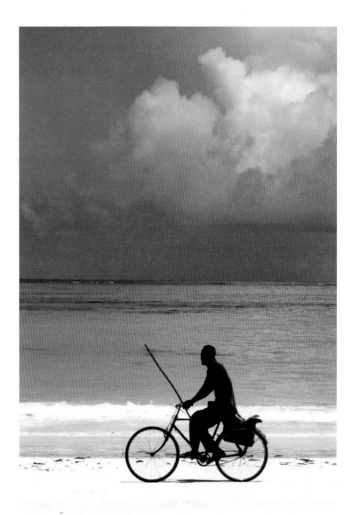

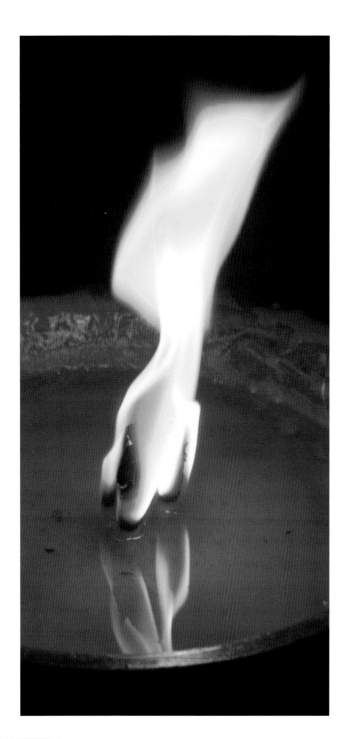

Pitta

This is the medium dosha, portrayed by the colour red, the force of heat and energy, linked with the sun that controls digestion and all biochemical processes in the body.

- Pitta types are evenly proportioned and of average height, a happy medium of the three doshas.

- They are confident and ambitious, and can be aggressively competitive.

- The dominant element is fire, then water.

- The seat of Pitta is the stomach and small intestine.

- A shared quality with Vata is lightness.

- Tastes that increase Pitta are sour, salty, pungent. Pitta types should avoid red meat.

- Tastes that pacify Pitta are sweet, astringent, bitter, cooling foods, especially salads, and also chicken, fish, tofu and mushrooms.

- The Pitta season is summer.

- Massage pressure should be moderate and consistent.

Characteristics of Pitta include:

- Strong appetite
- Tendency to sweat
- Frequent need to urinate
- Loose stools and tendency to diarrhoea
- Loud speech
- Interest in technical and scientific matters
- Care with money
- Tendency to jealousy
- Ambition and egotism
- Passionate and domineering sex drive
- Love of sport
- Interest in politics
- A love of luxury
- Dislike of heat

Health problems associated with Pitta include:

- Ulcers
- Digestive problems
- Gall bladder and liver problems
- Skin complaints
- Headaches

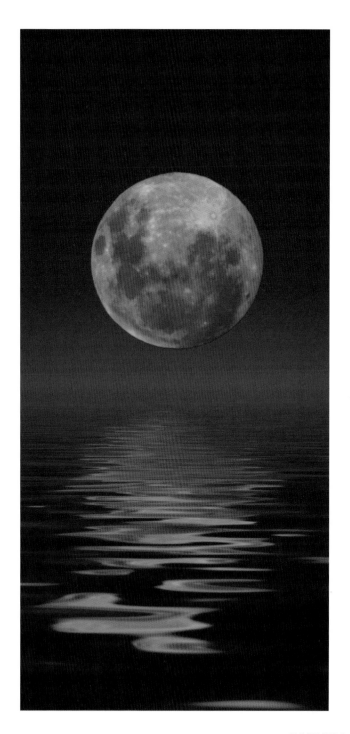

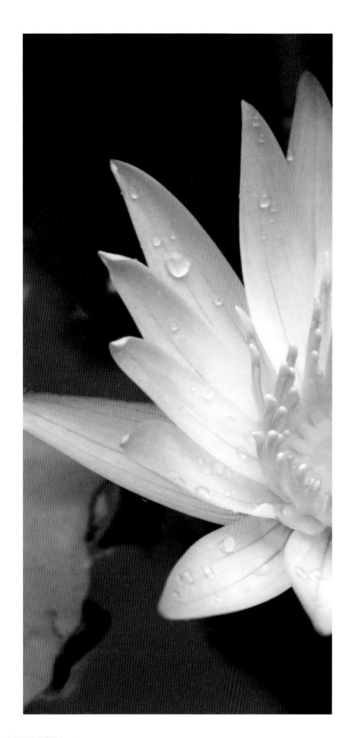

Kapha

This is the heaviest dosha, portrayed by the colour yellow. It is the force of water and tides and is influenced by the moon, the stabilising influence that controls fluid metabolism in the body.

- Kapha types are heavily built, lethargic, slow moving and physically strong.

- They are stable and patient, but inclined to possessiveness.

- The dominant element is earth, then water.

- The seat of Kapha is the lungs and stomach.

- A shared quality with Pitta is oiliness.

- Tastes that increase Kapha are sweet, sour, salty. Kapha types should avoid dairy produce.

- Tastes that pacify Kapha are pungent, bitter, astringent; hot and spicy food; apples and pears, also leaf vegetables, beans and lentils.

- The Kapha season is the mid-winter.

- Massage pressure should be deep and movements fast.

Characteristics of Kapha include:

- Moderate to sluggish appetite

- Heavy sweating

- Profuse but infrequent urination

- Large, soft stools

- Melodious speech

- Business-like approach

- Good memory

- Careful decision making

- Thrift and care with money - tendency to save and conserve

- Monogamy

- Lethargy and passivity

- A love of peace and quiet, and familiar places

- Love of good food

- Dislike of cold, damp conditions

Health problems associated with Kapha include:

- Hypertension

- Heart disease

- Circulatory disorders

- Diabetes

- Gall bladder problems

- Eczema

- Asthma

- Sinusitis

- Bronchitis

When all of these doshas are perfectly in balance in an individual, it means that all the systems and activities of mind and body are functioning at optimal levels; therefore, the individual enjoys perfect health. When one or more of these doshas goes out of balance, disorders result. To restore good health, the dosha that has become imbalanced needs to be restored to its original make-up in that specific individual.

Although Ayurveda is a complete system of medicine, and people turn to it for help in treating disorders, it is only as effective as the commitment from the client. Like all complementary medicine, the system is limited in its effectiveness: the client, before and after treatment, must lead a healthy lifestyle and address the cause of the physical and psychological harm being experienced.

The recommended Ayurvedic lifestyle is straightforward to follow and fits in with most modern life and work patterns. As with other complementary approaches, it aims to maintain and, where necessary, restore harmony of body, mind and spirit without resorting to drugs that often have adverse side-effects. It encourages calmness and discourages constant, frenetic activity. Body and mind benefit when individuals can adopt a meditative approach to life.

Stress is a widespread and serious modern problem, not least because it suffers from being 'fashionable'. It appears that there is now a tendency to blame everything on stress, coupled with a mindset that believes we have little control over its prevalence. The system of Ayurveda aims to challenge this mindset.

Similarly to other holistic approaches, the basis of Ayurveda is an approach that seeks to take a comprehensive account of all aspects of an individual's health and lifestyle. Unlike Western medicine, it does not divide the medical disciplines into specialities: this latter approach inevitably sees a 'condition' rather than a 'patient'.

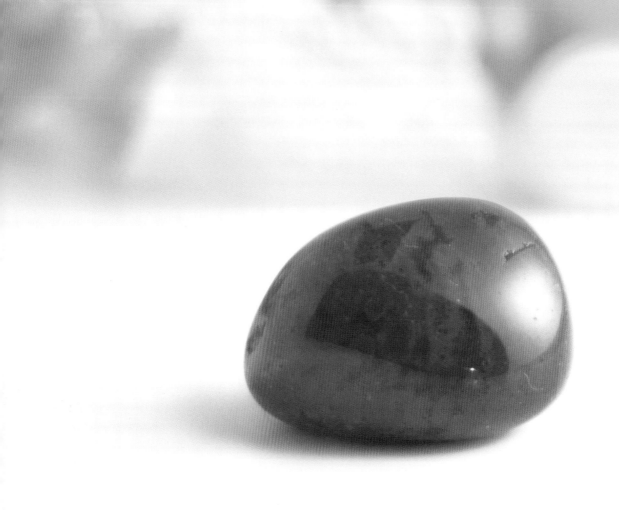

"The only thing that stands between a person and what they want from life is often the will to try it and the faith to believe it's possible"

Rich Devo

CRYSTALS

Crystals have been used throughout history for their healing qualities and beauty. From the Inuit of the Arctic to the Indians of the Amazon, shamanistic cultures throughout the world have valued precious and semi-precious gems for the magical and therapeutic qualities attributed to them. Crystals, particularly quartz crystals such as amethyst and rose quartz, are believed to possess healing 'life energy', storing and discharging this rather like a battery.

Healers believe the gems and crystals placed on and around clients can focus and enhance healing energies. Some suggest placing the crystals around the home to absorb negativity or improve the atmosphere, but they need to be washed regularly under cold running water and 'recharged' by placing then in direct sunlight or a full moon. It's suggested the uncut stones posses more energy than the polished stones – choose those you're drawn too and you won't go far wrong.

Many people believe that each stone emits a certain energy that can have a beneficial effect on our well-being. Does it work? Wear one, carry it with you, take it to bed and judge for yourself.

There are more than two hundred gem and mineral stones and essences, so this chapter will focus on the crystals that assist with skincare.

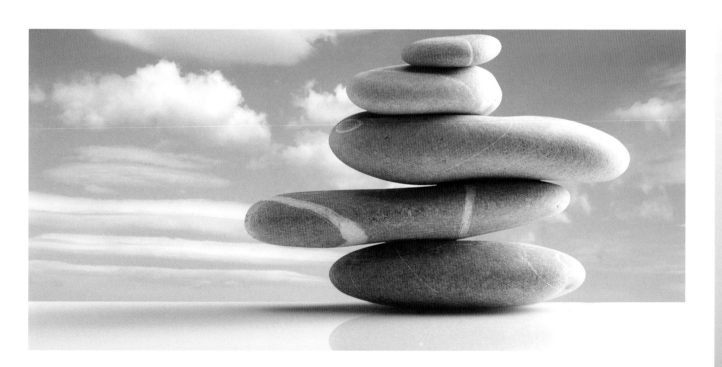

Amethyst - a very powerful aid to creative thinking, spiritual awareness and healing. Believed to combat insomnia. Strengthens the cleansing and eliminating organs and the immune system. An excellent cleanser for the blood.

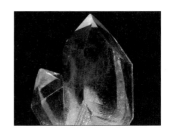

Ametrine - the entwined powers of amethyst and citrine make this unique stone, believed to be an exceptional blood cleanser and energiser. Helps to disperse toxins from the body and oxygenates the blood

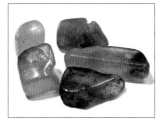

Bloodstone - can improve a sense of creativity, decision making and intuition. Said to help purify the blood and clear toxins. An immune stimulator, it stimulates the flow of lymph and the metabolic processes, purifies the blood and detoxifies the liver, intestines, kidneys, spleen and bladder. Regulates and supports blood flow and aids circulation. It reduces the formation of pus and neutralises over-acidification.

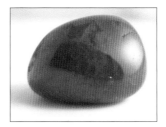

Carnelian - a good balancer, it connects you with your inner self, giving good concentration. Said to benefit the kidneys, lungs and liver. It stimulates the metabolism. Improves the absorption of vitamins and minerals and ensures a good supply of blood to organs and tissues.

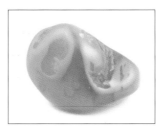

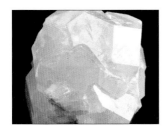

Fluorite/Pink Fluorite - this stone is believed to bring forth order from chaos, whilst uplifting and inducing relaxation. It is thought to fend off colds. Regenerates the skin and mucus membranes. Helps to heal the skin, removing blemishes and wrinkles.

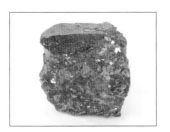

Hematite - enhances personal magnetism, will and courage. Believed to be beneficial for blood flow, stress and the nerves. It supports the kidneys in cleansing blood and tissue regeneration. Stimulates the absorption of iron and the formation of red blood cells.

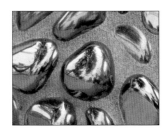

Rhodonite - a stimulating stone thought to be good for dispelling anxiety, encouraging generosity and providing a general feeling of well-being. Excellent as a wound healer that also relieves insect bites. It can reduce scarring.

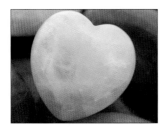

Rose Quartz - known as the 'love stone', it aids peacefulness and calm in relationships. Said to ease stress and tension and assist sleep. Strengthens the circulatory system and releases impurities from body fluids. Soothes burns and blistering and smoothes the complexion.

Snowflake Obsidian - a 'stone of purity' bringing balance to the body, mind and spirit. Said to be beneficial for the skin and veins, and improves circulation. The elixir is good for the skin and eyes.

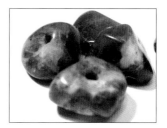

Sodalite - helps to calm and clear the mind, bring joy and relieve a heavy heart. Said to aid metabolism, it also cleanses the lymphatic system and organs, boosting the immune system. It cools fever, lowers blood pressure and stimulates the absorption of fluid in the body

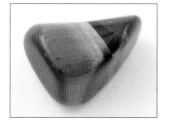

Tiger Eye - the 'confidence stone', inspiring brave but sensible behaviour. Believed to aid the entire digestive system. Heals the throat and reproductive organs. Emotionally balances the yin-yang and energises the emotional body. It alleviates depression and lifts moods

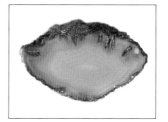

Turritella Agate - is believed to help in times of change, dispelling negative thoughts and relieving conditions of fatigue. Will stimulate the aura, eliminating and transforming negative energies. Can stimulate the digestive process to help relieve gastritis. Cleanses the lymphatic system and the pancreas. Strengthens blood vessels and heals skin disorders.

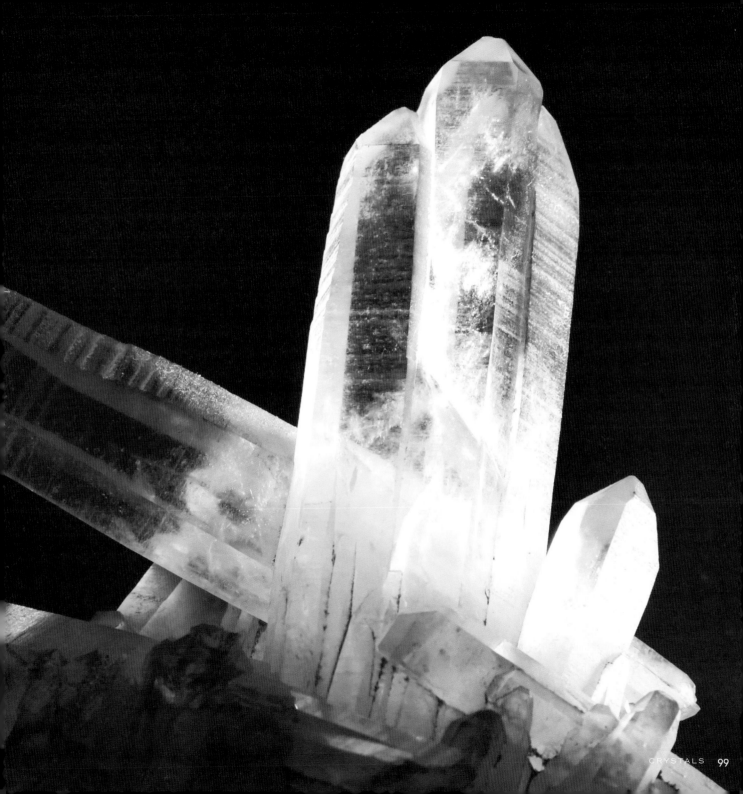

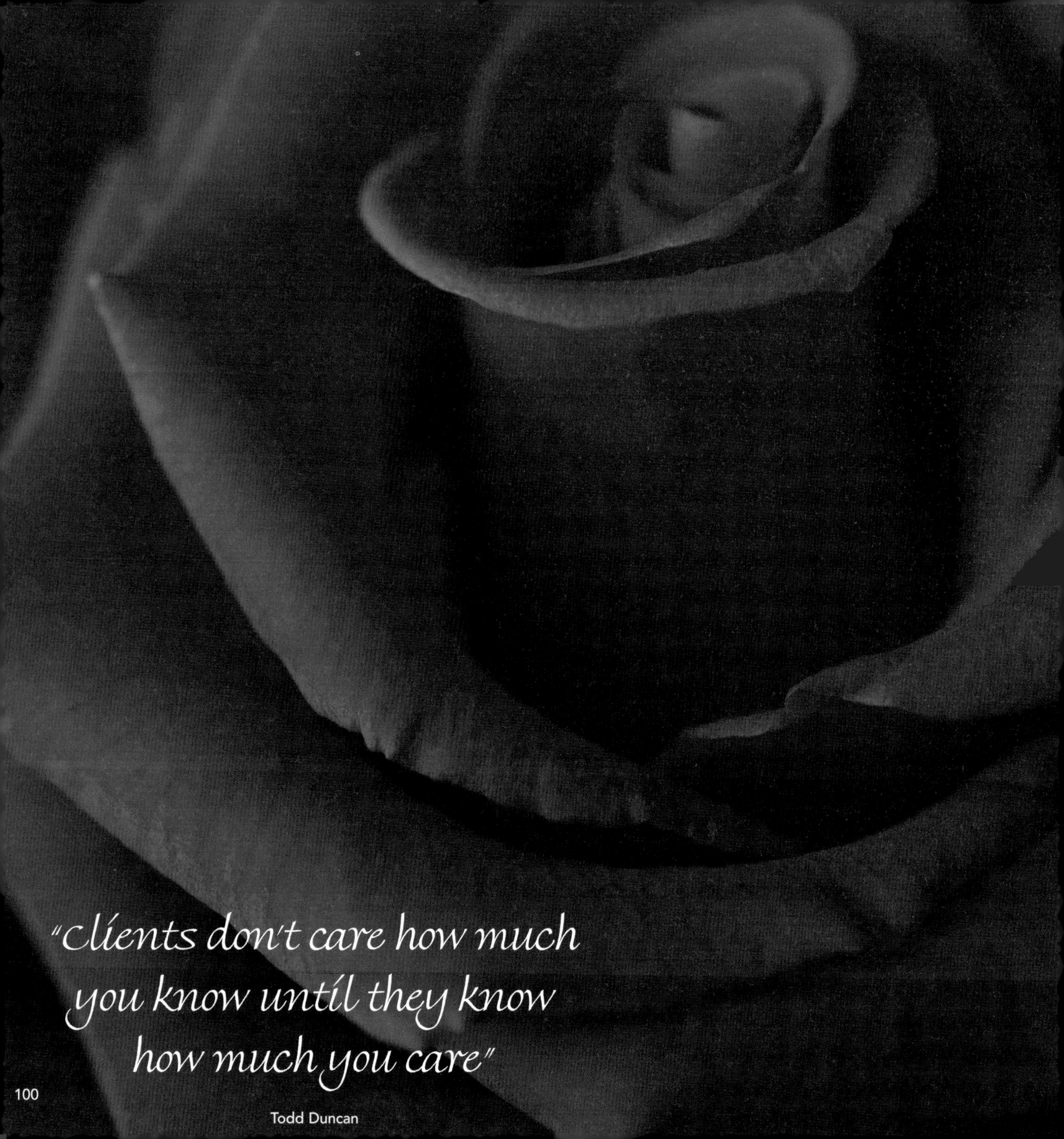

*"clients don't care how much
you know until they know
how much you care"*

Todd Duncan

ROMANCING THE CUSTOMER

The Key to Successful Retail Sales

The objective of this chapter is to share some of the approaches I have found successful for increasing retail sales in the spa and salon. Ultimately, each and every skincare therapist needs to develop a technique or an approach that feels right for them.

In my experience, both as a client and as a successful therapist, retail is all about giving a damn. It is absolutely nothing to do with 'flogging stuff' and everything to do with caring about each and every client who places themselves into your professional care.

In all retail arenas, there are individuals for whom sales just magically happen and those for whom sales remain something of an enigma. This chapter aims to enlighten the sales-enigma therapist and inspire the successful one. Whatever the case, I would love for every therapist to feel great about retail and every client to feel great about indulging in a little, but highly pleasurable, retail therapy.

Stop, Look and Listen

Having been responsible for selling anything from skincare to sheepskin coats, I have found there are two constants: a passion for the product and a sincere determination to delight the customer. Very early in my retail career, I was given a valuable piece of advice, and that was to use my eyes, ears and mouth in the ratio that God had provided. Therefore, trust what you see, listen, listen and listen some more, and only then share your observations.

This may all sound pretty obvious. In my experience, though, the listening part is skipped almost every time. This is where client care and retail sales are lost in a moment. The skill is to match the needs of the client with the best product or advice, and the only way to do this is to develop excellent listening skills. Although it can sometimes feel like you have to have the instincts of a detective with the skills of a mind-reader, effective listening really does mean the difference between a sale and the client leaving with nothing.

Develop a mentality that means you can let go of the outcome - work without an agenda. The second that you (or your manager) has an agenda, the sale will mysteriously disappear. Clients are not stupid and will recognise when they are being sold to rather than being genuinely helped and supported by a great therapist. You may disagree; perhaps they yield to your sales pitch and you get the sale, but I can guarantee you will lose the customer. They will no longer trust you and therefore won't book for more treatments or spa visits, so the short-term win has resulted in a long-term loss. The quote I hold in mind is that 'trust takes a lifetime to build but is lost in a heartbeat'.

Always be sincere, genuine and full of integrity when recommending products to your client. Sometimes this means recommending a product or service you don't sell. My experience is that clients will be so thrilled with your honesty and integrity, they will recommend you whenever they can.

When Do I Start to Retail?

The second you greet the client! Even with regular clients, make a habit of bringing into your consciousness everything you notice about them the moment you meet. Are they slumped in the chair looking totally frazzled, or are they looking alert and vital? Do they look anxious or self-conscious, or do they appear at ease and full of anticipation? What's the condition of their skin? Is it inflamed, sallow, dry, oily? Trust what your eyes are telling you, then use this information to act as a silent cue to how they are feeling and let this shape your approach during their treatment.

For the anxious client, you need to discover what it is that is making them feel uncomfortable. It may be that they have never had a facial treatment before. Or perhaps the treatment was a gift voucher given by a 'thoughtful' friend or loved one but is, in fact, the client's idea of hell. For this client, everything you ask will be seen as a potential 'trap' for them to fall into, that all you're interested in is selling them something they don't need, so they are full of suspicion about your motives.

Whatever the reason, you need to put them at ease as quickly as possible. Begin by introducing yourself (and understand that they will forget this information in an instant!). On the journey through to the treatment room, get your nervous client used to answering your questions by making general enquiries about their journey. Did they find you easily? Are they enjoying the weather? Do they know anyone who's benefited from a treatment with you before. What is the thing they are most looking forward to today. Do all this before you've reached the treatment room. This helps them become familiar and relaxed about answering your questions

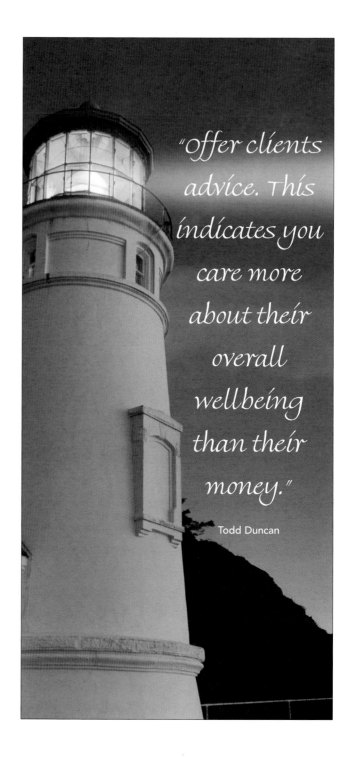

"Offer clients advice. This indicates you care more about their overall wellbeing than their money."

Todd Duncan

so that, when you begin to enquire about their skincare routines and concerns, responding to you doesn't feel like a trap, it just feels natural.

~ Consultation ~

This is where you become a skincare detective. As a general rule, I 'store' the information gathered when we first meet in reception and I use this to inform what I say during the consultation. This needs to be an affirmation of what you have already noticed; there should be no big surprises.

Best practice is for the majority of the consultation card to be completed by the client on their arrival or whilst waiting to be collected. This saves time and allows you to make more detailed enquiries once they are settled and comfortable on the treatment couch. If you feel passionately that a client should not complete this independently, it is probably a good idea to train the reception staff or spa assistants to do this on your behalf.

I have found that, once in the treatment room, questions that focus exclusively on the client are the ones which help to create feelings of trust and genuine understanding. The alternative means your client feels like they are on a conveyer belt and you won't stay in business very long!

At all costs, avoid asking questions like a pilot's check-list; instead inject some compassion and understanding. You could try one of the following questions.

- I notice from your consultation that you have sensitive skin. Can you tell me more about this?

- Describe for me your current skincare routine. For example, do you like the sensation of water on your face, or do you use cotton wool to cleanse?

- I see you are concerned about dry skin. Do you find it is like that all year round?

- Is time an issue? Perhaps you have more time in the evening?

- I see you use facial wipes. What is it about using this product that you find works?

- When was the last time your skin looked and felt its absolute best?

~ Making negative judgements ~

Never let the client feel you are judging them; nothing will alienate you faster than a negative judgment, however well-intentioned you are. You are the professional therapist, supported by years of training and experience. The client may be well-informed but they are still susceptible to the persuasive marketing techniques employed by cosmetic companies, who are largely playing to our vulnerabilities and insecurities about a perpetually youthful appearance and the banishing of wrinkles.

These messages are highly seductive and can prove irresistible to even the most well-informed individual. The cry from most clients when they learn the truth is 'how can the manufacturers get away with making these claims?' In fact, manufacturers often suggest 'benefits' rather than making an outright claim.

So a client is judged negatively by you for buying a product, possibly as a result of persuasive marketing, only to learn that the product is damaging their skin. The client is going to be feeling especially ticked off; don't add insult to injury by giving them a lecture.

When clients are describing their favourite products or skincare routines, watch your body language or non-verbal communication. These include:

- Raised eyebrows

- Sharp in-take of breath

- Pursing the lips

- Squinting the eyes

- Frowning

- Tutting

I also feel strongly that you need to work with their 'given'. This can include poor nutrition, not drinking enough water, unmanaged stress, smoking and drinking too much alcohol, coffee or caffeine-loaded drinks. Instead, encourage them to protect their skin from the negative effects of these lifestyle choices by using products rich in antioxidants such as vitamins A, C and E or bioflavonoids and so on. It will no doubt come as a refreshing change not to receive a lecture about the damage they are doing to themselves, most of which they know already.

I know my view is a controversial one. However, my own feeling about poor lifestyle choices is that if the fear of heart attack, high blood pressure and cancer isn't enough to motivate clients to change, ageing wrinkles and a dull complexion are unlikely to shock them into doing something! Gentle encouragement, mixed with some humour and a dash of empathy is the best recipe for empowering clients to change.

~ Opening the sale ~

Or should I say 'Starting the cleanse process'... Limit the amount of questions you ask to maybe three or four before you start the cleanse procedure, and always sit facing your client when you do this, never behind them.

From the consultation, you will have identified what kind of cleanser your client prefers. If they like a facial wash, use a wash-off cleanser. If they prefer cleansing milk and cotton wool, guess what, use cleansing milk!

From a retail perspective, it is pointless using a product on a client if it isn't something you could introduce as an alternative to what they currently use. Likewise, if they have dry skin and you know their current choice of cleanser is responsible for this, use the cleanse process to communicate your thoughts and demonstrate the alternative. Try the following and see which approach feels right for you.

Begin with 'You mentioned concerns over your...' (this could be their dry, oily, sensitive, wrinkled skin... be informed and share your knowledge to the benefit of the client.)

Add to this statements such as:

- You might like to consider...

- Have you thought about...

- Perhaps you might like to...

- Many of my clients are unaware that...

Share your knowledge of ingredients with comments such as:

- Restricting facial wipes as a cleanser to when time is tight...

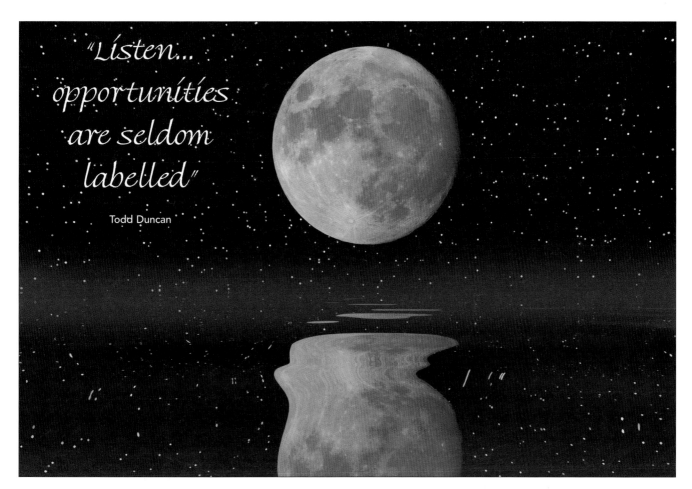

> *"Listen...*
> *opportunities*
> *are seldom*
> *labelled"*
>
> Todd Duncan

- The toner you use contains SD alcohol...

- Your cleanser contains colourants...

- The fragranced moisturiser you currently use...

End with:

- I am sure, having worked with your skin that...

- Many of my clients have found replacing...

- You will probably find the... is not helping the problem

- You will probably find... is the problem

The cleanse process is where much of the observations and advice you offer needs to take place. This acts as a prompt to the client and gives them 'food for thought' during the remainder of the treatment (known as creating the need). I confine my comments to what I see and feel, linking it back to their initial concerns at every opportunity.

The cleanse procedure is the start of the retail process for two reasons: this is the first opportunity

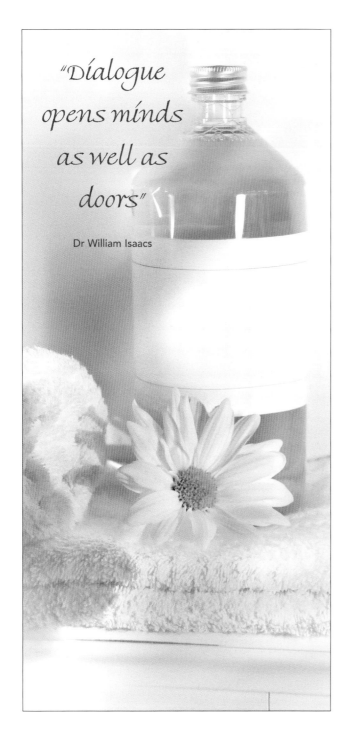

"Dialogue opens minds as well as doors"

Dr William Isaacs

you will have had to touch your client's skin; and it is the least quiet time of the facial (running water, different textures, hands stopping and starting, client just starting to get comfortable and so on), so your comments are less likely to disturb your client's relaxation and may even become a welcome distraction.

~ Regular clients ~

Try to avoid making any assumptions about your regular clients; this can make the difference between them feeling taken care of, or being taken for granted. They have needs and expectations as well. Obviously you will have a slightly more relaxed and informal approach with regular clients, and clearly you don't need to ask them if they found you easily, but you do need to guard against falling into conversations that have nothing to do with them or why they are seeing you.

Have a little catch-up from their last visit, but then the focus must be on them and their skin, their health and their well-being. This was once described to me as 'chit-chat not clap-trap'. In fact, one of the greatest threats to the success of your retail sales with regular clients is to assume that they will ask for products rather than appreciate a prompt or two from you. They won't ask and they will buy their products somewhere else, I guarantee it.

During my retail training workshops, one of the most impassioned complaints from therapists working with regular clients is that retail is harder because 'they don't need anything' or 'they've got everything already'. Conversely, spa therapists always make a similar complaint, except that they can't retail because the client is only there for a day or two.

Both are lame excuses.

As someone who has been a client far longer than I've been a therapist, I know I appreciate it (and subsequently spend money) when my regular therapist reminds me my cleanser is likely to be running out and that I may need to take some with me today. I also appreciate being made to feel individual and special by the spa therapist who takes the time to recommend something because 'I see from your consultation that you weren't sleeping well' or whatever. Both instances are about giving a damn.

With regular clients, there are any number of computer software packages that can track customer buying patterns, treatment preferences and all sorts of personal details. You could also use the good old pen and paper method by recording client information on their consultation card. It doesn't need to be complicated, but it does need to be done. How else are you going to remember each client's purchases?

~ Closing the sale ~

Once the massage and mask procedure is completed, it is time to start bringing the client gently back to planet earth. I begin by quietly but animatedly describing what differences I notice with their skin. This must be genuine. If you stay with the premise of believing what you see, you can take this one stage further and communicate what you see.

Try the following for ways of doing this:

- One product that made a real difference today was... (often the exfoliator or mask)

- If you do nothing else, consider introducing...

- It's interesting. I noticed when I used the... it was amazing how quickly your skin responded

- Your skin tone is far more even now

- Your skin looks smooth now

- Your skin is glowing/clear/fresh

- You look radiant/relaxed/less stressed

- Have you thought about...

I tend to focus on the one product that will make a difference to the client, and this goes right back to the quality of the consultation. If you don't know what the focus is for the client, you are pitching in the dark. You have to understand their concern or need before you can offer a solution.

Once you are taking a glass of water or herbal tea to a client, enquire about how their skin feels - we know they are going to be feeling wonderful, they've just enjoyed a great treatment from a great therapist. What you need to get the client to do is focus on the benefits of what your treatment has done to their skin.

Try the following for closing the sale:

- Having seen how wonderfully your skin has responded to...

- Having seen how much smoother your skin is now...

- Really pleased you agree your skin has become softer. This will be the...

- The exfoliator is perfect for your concerns about the dry skin you mentioned...

- X product has made such a difference to your skin, you can't leave without it!

Another common concern is when the client asks the often dreaded question: 'How much does it cost?' To get the main focus off the price (because this is rarely, if ever, the real reason why people don't buy), respond with the following question: 'Just so that I can help you best, can I ask you a couple of questions first...?' Then bring the focus back to their initial concern.

In short, ask a question (clarify and focus), wait for the client's reply (affirmation) and respond with empathic emphasis (final focusing of the mind).

- How itchy is your dry skin... ? So it sounds like it really gets you down...

- How much of a problem is an oily T-zone... ? Sounds like it badly affects your confidence...

- What is it about your breakouts that bothers you... ? From what you've described, I can see how that would leave you feeling upset...

Hopefully this gives you the idea. After this, go ahead and tell your client the price. I never hold it back, never have an apologetic or astonished tone and always deliver this in a matter-of-fact way. I have found that this way of responding is a highly effective way of getting the focus off the price.

Negative Feelings about Retail

When working with therapists, I believe firmly that each and every person has their own style and this is the key to their success with repeat bookings, retail sales and client referrals. If you recognise yourself as one of the many therapists who find retailing tough, take time to discover:

- What it feels like to retail. Some therapists describe how their mouth goes dry just at the thought of selling a product; others describe sweaty palms, verbal blackouts or, worse still, gabbling uncontrollably! Others get butterflies, flushed faces, weak knees and any number of awful feelings. Think about where you feel your negativity and anxiety.

These are all indicators of stress, and the great news is that this can be easily overcome.

Next examine your:

- Thought process, prior to and during the retail conversation. For the majority, it has to do with feeling you're being asked to do something you don't feel comfortable with. Or perhaps you fear that the client will say 'No'. Other favourite cop-outs are 'We're therapists, not sales assistants', or 'I'm a holistic therapist and I don't sell'. And then there's the 'last resort' excuse for any therapist: 'I don't have time'.

Finally, adopt:

- A solution to these points. Every single point against retailing from a skincare therapist can be met with a reason to retail from therapists working holistically and professionally. The success is to discover what your natural, personal style is and to practise this until retail conversations start to happen instinctively.

There is often a 'Top 3' to the reasons therapists give for not wanting to retail; here is a selection of the most common of these.

- **Feeling guilty**. The most heartfelt and frequently cited reason given by therapists for not wanting to retail is that they feel guilty. What do you have to feel guilty about? If the client doesn't want to buy products, they won't. It's that simple. Your responsibility is to recommend and match the best products for their concerns; if they then decide to decline the chance to make a difference, so be it. They will still appreciate the fact that you cared and took the time to offer great advice. Providing you maintain your integrity, and only ever offer appropriate advice, you have nothing to feel guilty about. Not responding to a client's concern or failing to address a problem you have identified - now that's something to feel guilty about.

- **Ripping people off**. Another fear expressed by therapists is that they are 'ripping off the client'. If the products you're retailing do what they're meant to (and why would you stock them if they don't?), you're only ripping people off if you're not telling the truth, you're being insincere or you're introducing something they don't need. Always try to hold in mind that clients will pick up on your body language, so if you're feeling uncomfortable or uneasy, it will make them suspicious of anything you say. Practise the skill of retailing in the same way as you would practise any new skill. Think about how awkward you felt when you first started as a therapist; retail is no different. Psychologists say that we need to do something about twenty times before it becomes habit - so persevere and enjoy the benefits.

- **Don't know if they have the money**. A further reason given by therapists is the apprehension about the amount of money a client may have spent already on the treatment. 'So what?' is my response. A client coming for a treatment is there to be taken care of AS WELL AS to enjoy a great treatment. Thinking that the treatment is enough is a mistake: part of what the client is paying for is your expertise and professional advice. I used to get so frustrated if I had a treatment with a therapist who didn't bother to offer me any

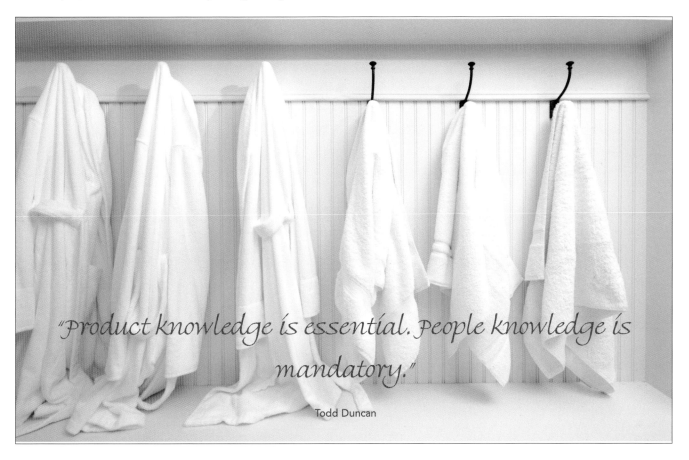

"Product knowledge is essential. People knowledge is mandatory."

Todd Duncan

advice. Don't misunderstand me, they gave a fabulous treatment; they just didn't help me feel taken care of. For me, its the equivalent of visiting the dentist for a check-up and the dental surgeon not commenting on my dental health. There's nothing wrong with the check-up, that's what you paid for, but it's as though they can't be bothered with anything beyond this. As a therapist, you can not assume anything about the client's disposable income; irrespective of how pushy you imagine you're being, a client won't buy if they don't want to.

Summary

As a professional skincare therapist, it may be helpful to hold in mind the following points.

- The advice you offer is not for your benefit.

- You are offering your professional opinion, based on years of hard work and study.

- The advice you offer needs to be objective, genuine and sincere.

- You are being helpful, not pushy.

- The client is paying for your professional care and knowledge.

- You have entered into a caring profession. This means you are failing to fulfil your responsibility as a therapist by not explaining solutions to their skincare concerns.

The skill of retailing is largely about having a natural conversation with another person, which at its heart has their concerns and your solutions. Great retailing is done with passion, honesty and enthusiasm; it certainly shouldn't be boring, stressful or dull!

For the uninitiated, retail needs to be practised to enable you to find the perfect style for you. Mine is a mix of child-like cheekiness and professional authority. You need to find yours and evolve with it. Be adaptable: each client will respond to you in a different way. Some will demand a more formal approach, some want more technical information, whilst others want to have fun and gentle persuasion to treat themselves - the 'go on, you know you want to' factor.

Above all else, enjoy the process. Retail is meant to be fun!

Useful Questions

Here are some questions that you may find useful to ask your clients. They will help you to become a successful skincare detective and retailer.

What

What can I help you with today?

What products are you using now?

What results do you want to achieve?

What consistency do you like for your moisturiser?

What kind of product are you looking for?

What problems are you experiencing today?

What made you select our spa/salon?

What have you enjoyed most about the experience today?

What products do you need to restock with today?

What results do you expect from today's treatment?

When

When was the last time your skin was at its absolute best?

When did you last change your skincare routine?

When do you use a mask/exfoliating product etc?

When do you apply your eye cream?

When was the last time you had a facial?

When do you think you'll run out of your existing product?

Where

Where have you had a treatment before?

Where are you applying your eye cream?

Where do you store your products?

How

How much of product X do you have?

How do you apply your moisturiser?

How many do you want?

How about a change?

How would you like to be the first to try this?

How does your skin feel after cleansing?

How long after cleansing does your skin show oil?

How do you cleanse your skin?

How would you like your skin to feel?

Why

Why do you want to change?

Why are you hesitating?

Why do you believe the product isn't working?

Why don't you give it a try?

Why don't we book you in whilst we have appointments?

Who

Who recommended you to use our salon/spa?

Whose product are you using?

Who told you about product X?

Which

Which time would be most convenient?

Which product do you prefer?

Other useful starters for questions include:

- Do you prefer?
- Are you?
- Have you?
- Would you?
- Will you?

Little yeses add up, so use these questions during the treatment:

- Does that make sense?
- Is that alright?
- Is this fair?
- Would you prefer?
- Are you comfortable/happy with what we've done so far?
- Do you like the feel?
- Does the product feel great?
- You can tell the difference now, can't you?

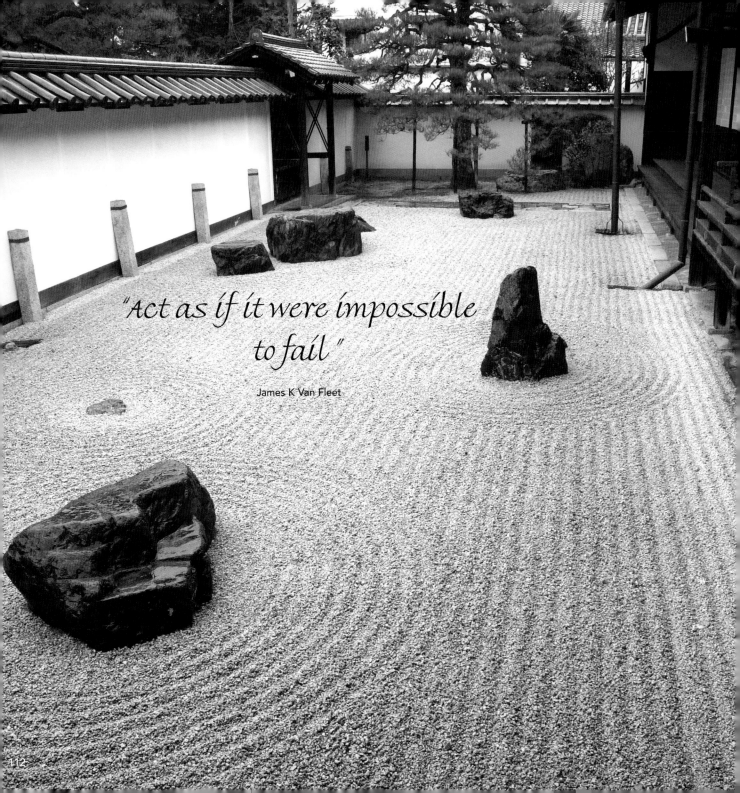

"Act as if it were impossible to fail"

James K Van Fleet

VISUAL MERCHANDISING

The objective of this chapter is to share some of the proven methods of merchandising that will have a positive effect on the retail sales and profitability of your business. I believe ignoring the retail presentation in your salon or spa could be a sign of commercial insanity; the potential to create straightforward, easy profit must not be underestimated. Read on and learn some of the subtle skills used to seduce customers into indulging in a little, but highly pleasurable, retail therapy.

Great visual merchandising is about a passion for detail, a critical eye for standards and an understanding of your sales environment. Its power is phenomenal, its effect well proven. It defines brand delivery, creates a better retail experience for your client and a brighter future for your business. The aim is to drive retail sales and increase your profitability.

In any environment, visual merchandising is the equivalent of having a member of staff working for you around the clock: they never take a break, never have a day off sick, don't need a holiday and never lose their passion and enthusiasm for the products they are selling!

The Masters of Merchandising

Supermarkets are incredibly successful when it comes to seducing us into making purchases we hadn't planned - and we don't ever resent it or feel conned in the process. You have the same capacity to create these seductive messages, and in spas and salons I believe you can stimulate the senses even more successfully than in giant supermarkets.

The success of supermarkets is due to their talent for manipulating our senses. To begin with, colour and smell help to invite us into an environment, so this is where the fruit and vegetable section is located. It makes no logical sense since all of the hard goods, like washing powder and baked beans, will potentially crush the soft produce, like grapes and apples. The reason they do it is because the fruit and veg section provides an excellent variety of colour and fragrance, and also gets us relaxed and engaged in the buying process through our sense of touch.

Good retailers know that the more relaxed we are, the more time we spend in their shops, and more time means more opportunities to tempt us into buying more than we planned. The key to getting people to spend longer in a store depends on how comfortable and enjoyable the experience is.

'Dwell time' is directly correlated with sales, so if you create a more pleasant environment and increase dwell time, sales rise.

Effective merchandising helps people feel confident and therefore good about buying into your brand, it communicates how great your products are and it means your customer doesn't have to work hard in the process. Make no assumptions about the amount of time people have to browse: your merchandising needs to be clear, easy to navigate and effortless to shop from.

Getting it right is no longer a luxury, it's an essential driver to delivering brand and financial success for your business.

In the beauty and spa retail business, you now have to compete in an environment that is becoming increasingly saturated, and you also have to consider the threat of web-based shopping as the preferred option for many cash-rich, time-poor consumers. The UK has the highest number of on-line sales, up to 50% compared to a worldwide average of 30%, and this figure is growing.

One area where the Internet cannot compete with you is in providing a sensory shopping experience. Appealing to the emotions is one of the things that retailers do best. People enter the retail area to be seduced, and appealing to more than one sense is the key to that seduction.

The traditional experience of shopping in the spa is becoming far more demanding, and your role is to romance the customer by employing some subtle skills to seduce them into indulging in a little, but highly pleasurable retail therapy

Acoustics in the Retail Area

Psycho-acoustics or, more simply, what we hear in the retail environment is phenomenally powerful. This is one sense that is often ignored or completely bypassed in the planning and design of salons and

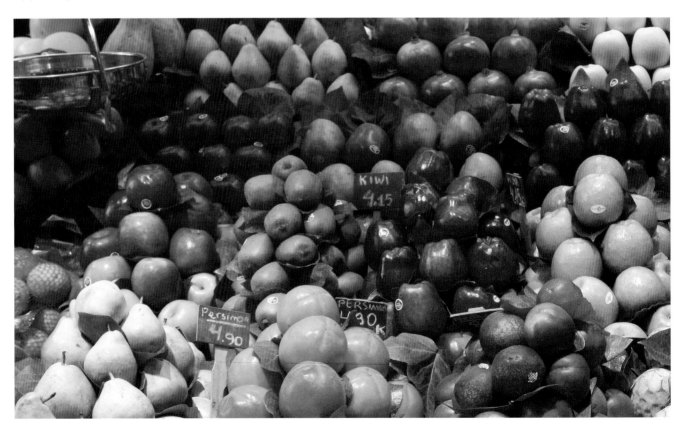

spas. Not just in the retail area but throughout the reception, relaxation areas, treatment rooms and changing areas.

So powerful is the area of psycho-acoustics that it can and does affect how we respond in any given environment. In restaurants it has been used to make us eat more quickly, or more slowly, order specific dishes or wines and raise our perception of the financial worth.

In the retail environment, there have been experiments conducted with music in the wine section of supermarkets. For one week, German music was played and the sales of German wines tracked. The following week, French music was played and, likewise, French wine sales tracked. Both experiments showed a significant increase in sales of the wine where the corresponding music was playing.

In a college refectory, classical music was played for several weeks, followed by a student survey. The perception based on nothing other than the music being played was that the environment was believed to be more exclusive. It's worth noting that sales increased - clearly, classical music encourages more spending!

Many fast food and deli bars play faster, louder music at lunchtime. This way, we're encouraged to eat more quickly and deterred from dwelling for too long. Result? They can serve more covers and take more money.

The outcomes are amazing for such a subtle change in the environment, and of course we're almost totally unaware of these effects. Take time to consider what kind of music you have playing and what it is saying about your brand. What is the sound of your brand? What are your clients' perceptions of your brand based upon the music they are being exposed to? It could be the thing that makes an immediate, simple and profitable impact on the profitability of your business.

The Red Thread

The way to create a constant, clear and informative retail message is to identify any 'show case' opportunities that may exist in your environment, and then use these to maximum effect.

Such 'show case' areas are vital for creating a consistent message for the visiting client - a virtual red-thread - all of which strengthen your brand authority by communicating who you are, and what you do, in a style that is consistent and comprehensive.

This can be achieved by the careful and deliberate positioning of products and images to convert a client's want into a need. This is fundamental to all of the decisions we make when deciding to part with our hard-earned cash.

Clients and customers need to know not only what it is they are looking at, but what it is for, why it is great for them, and where can they buy it. Countless times we are exposed to images and displays that look good but don't tell the complete story. This is a missed opportunity.

~ Visual communication ~

Everything you expose customers to must help them understand which is the right product for them. Clarity in communication is the key to successful retailing. We are bombarded with thousands of messages every day so care is needed to ensure that your message is eye-catching and highly seductive. The message being communicated must be consistent and clear. This ensures you maintain credibility, authority and customer confidence. Consistency is persuasive and commercially successful, and helps to produce great visual merchandising that says 'you know you want to' rather than 'look but don't touch'. It is a genuine way of letting people know how great your brand, your products and your company are.

Emotional Decisions

We are emotionally driven and almost all retail purchases are made emotionally, not intellectually. Many decisions to buy retail products are made, or can be heavily influenced, in the environment you create in the relaxation area, the reception, treatment room and finally the retail area itself. If we only visited retail stores or the spa retail area when we needed to buy something, and if once there, we bought only what we needed, the UK economy would collapse.

Your clients are susceptible to impressions and information; you need to ensure the impressions they receive are the ones you intended.

As described, we all buy on emotion supported by logic, so your retail merchandising needs to inform and excite rather than confuse and overwhelm. It has a powerful impact on our senses and your profits. Don't let the reason for lost retail sales be because the retail merchandising is cluttered and confusing.

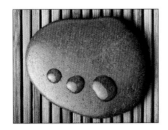
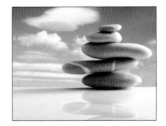
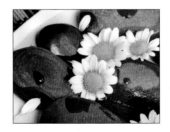
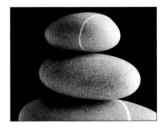

One last point on emotional reactions is the amount of time and effort a customer has to 'invest' before they are able to buy something. Many salons and spas lock their retail products behind glass. Inevitably this means the client not only has to ask your permission to buy something, but they also have to wait for someone to be free to unlock the cabinet, and then process the sale. It is worth holding in mind that, when customers are made to wait, their impression of your overall service plunges, irrespective of how great the experience has been up to this point.

Open Merchandising

To liberate the retail area, it's necessary to consider open merchandising versus closed merchandising. It's hard to overemphasise the importance of open merchandising in the spa and salon. This is rather a dramatic departure from the current trend of keeping everything locked behind glass, but a critical one nevertheless. Keeping merchandise behind locked cabinets guarantees that purchases are being prohibited. You can have the best product range in the world, with the most seductive merchandising displays, but if the client can't pick things up, it's a complete waste. If clients are unable to experience the product, they just won't buy.

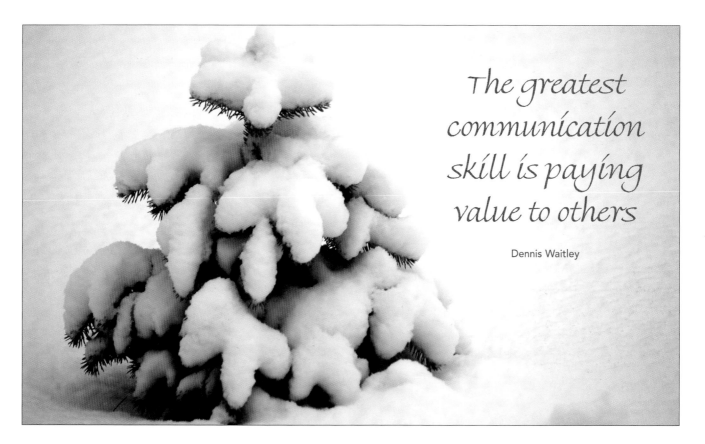

The greatest communication skill is paying value to others

Dennis Waitley

Clients buy things today more than ever on aroma and touch. We want to be blissed out by the fragrance, we want to know how it will feel on our skin. Although a client may have experienced the products during a treatment, the key is in reminding themselves how fabulous the products are by touching and smelling the products themselves. They won't have had the opportunity to participate in the product themselves because you, the therapist, applied it. Now its their turn. In retailing, the 'possession' or sensory experience of a product is the critical issue. Once a client has the product in their hand, they become emotionally connected. Paying for it then becomes a trivial point.

Tester stands are fabulous if positioned as close to the retail shelves as possible, but it can still require a degree of determination to actually make a purchase once a decision to buy something has been made. Nobody wants to wait whilst the receptionist finds the key, opens the cabinet and then hovers over your shoulder whilst you decide if you want to buy something else. I can't tell you how many times I have seen frustrated spa customers searching vainly for a member of staff to unlock the cabinet.

Selling is the main reason for stocking homecare products in the salon and the spa. So make them as accessible as you can. Countless times I see products locked away in dark cupboards. It's almost as though the decision to retail a particular brand somehow turns the stockist into a secret agent. We don't share the fabulous products on offer but assume the client will ask if they want something. They won't!

Making retail products as available as possible also creates an opportunity to up-sell and create link-sales. We need to be able to compare one product against another, otherwise we're limited to taking only what we're aware of. There is no opportunity to tempt ourselves with additional or complementary products. We need to take advantage of the unique opportunity we have to educate our clients about skincare, along with the need to communicate benefits. This means many will spend more than they had intended.

Another aspect of merchandising is to create logical adjacencies - the placing of one item next to another to create interest and increase the average spend. This is the major part of what adjacencies can deliver, namely add-on sales. Sometimes this is just the usual till-point 'impulse buy', but add-on sales can take place anywhere that homecare products are available. I believe spas and salons under-estimate this potential and their retail businesses suffer as a result. Specially created impulse purchases or promotional offers typically have a high profit margin, and they can make the difference between a salon that just gets by and one that prospers.

Making merchandise inaccessible damages your business in other ways, too. There is a fine balance between making something beautiful but precious and untouchable: you allow the client to like what they see but stop them from getting involved with the product. This is precisely what you don't want in a retail area where the objective is to encourage people to pick things up and take things home.

Customers have become accustomed to retailing environments where everything is accessible and on open display, with great promotional material giving them all the information they need. I don't know about you, but I always assume something is expensive if the retailer hasn't priced a product, and

I certainly won't ask. Firstly, it requires effort and, secondly, the fear is that it is out of my price bracket and I don't want to look a fool.

Much of the reluctance by spa managers and salon owners to throw open the locked door of the retail cabinets is the fear of people pinching the products. This is, sadly, a fact of retail life and so needs to be built onto the depreciation line on your profit and loss statements. It is, however, not all misery. To begin with, the up-turn in retail sales more than compensates for the loss from theft. If it didn't, we wouldn't have successful retailers on the high street.

There are also any number of security cameras that can be installed cost effectively, which act as effective deterrents. However, my belief and experience has shown that the most effective deterrent to shrinkage or theft from the retail area is to ensure all staff acknowledge the presence of every customer. This has a wonderful way of welcoming a genuine customer and is a very effective way of letting a potential thief know you've seen them. This can be a simple 'hello' or can be a direct comment about the product they are looking at.

As a slight deviation at this point, I make a solemn appeal that no one ever greets a customer with 'Hello, can I help you?' it is just so unimaginative, is almost always met with a 'No' from the customer and shows no enthusiasm for the product or your brand.

Customer Profile and Stunning Windows

This may sound like an obvious comment, but you need to know who your customer is in order to retail successfully. This not only involves decisions about the products you stock but also about where you position them.

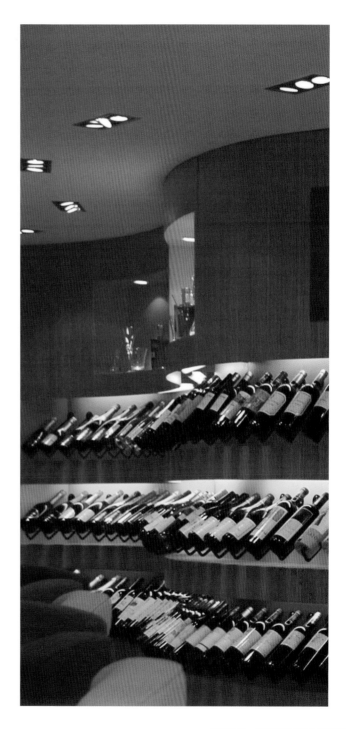

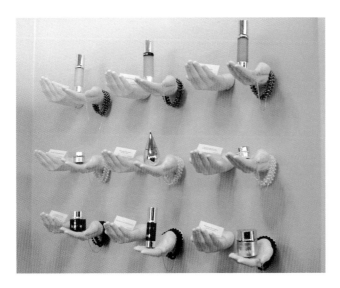

High-street salons and urban day spas need to use every available opportunity to capture the imagination of passing trade. No matter how strong your existing spa or salon brand, sooner or later you'll face competitors who do what you do, only better. Today's clients expect more, and there are enlightened spa and salon brands out there that will meet those expectations and reap the financial rewards. You need to ensure your brand is one of them.

The investment in hiring the professional services of a visual merchandising specialist will pay for itself ten-fold in the battle to stay ahead of your competitors. Window displays and internal cabinets need to communicate your retail and promotional message, and using a visual merchandiser will ensure you create window campaigns that have high impact and are memorable.

Spa brands can look vulnerable because of poor brand delivery, whilst the best companies are investing greater amounts to exceed their clients needs and expectations. The promotional or product message needs to be big and bold and short and simple, otherwise it's lost. Marketing messages in the window need to be read in an instant, no more than two or three words. Studies have shown that, on average, signs get less than two seconds' exposure per client. That's not many words.

Use humour and charm to delight the client, making your windows not only a commercial success but a critical necessity in defining brand delivery.

Use your promotions to build a little visual anticipation. With the promotional signage, first you need to get a client's attention. Once you've done that, you have to present your message in a clear, logical fashion - with a beginning, middle and ending. People will then have an opportunity to absorb the information a little at a time and in the right sequence. You have to capture their attention first otherwise nothing that follows will register. Too much information too soon and they become overloaded and give up. Finally, if you confuse them they will ignore the message altogether.

Repetition is critical to the success of promotional messages: several different messages, saying different things, will result in confusion. This means you lose credibility, authority and customer confidence and miss out on increased sales and profitability.

Day spas benefit from being able to drip feed their promotional messages by using several different locations throughout the spa. To achieve repeated and informative messages, the promotion needs to start at the spa reception desk and follow through to the treatment room, out into the relaxation area, ending with a strong and easy-to-find presentation in the retail area. This is the retail equivalent of a treasure hunt!

Tips for successful merchandising

- Keep smaller items just below or just above eye level - it is pointless merchandising them any lower or higher because customers will not stretch to reach up and they rarely, if ever, bend down to look at products.

- Larger items are better merchandised on lower shelves - visually it will look better and it is easier for clients to view big items at this height.

- Merchandise products in the sequence you might use them - cleanse, tone, moisturise or shower, bath and candles - this increases the likelihood of link purchases being made.

- Allocate more space to your best-selling products - this might mean merchandising them in more than one place.

- Link products together to create impulse purchases - cleansers with exfoliators or face serums with masks and so on.

- Position demand lines in the easy-to-reach areas or hot spots; never make it difficult to find your top 10 selling products.

- Remember that eye level is buy level - this is the best spot for the top 10 selling products

- Centre and centre right of the eye level shelf is the optimum space for creating sales.

- Position products that clients will need more time to browse and study away from busy and congested areas - people will not tolerate being bumped into.

- See your 'store' through the eyes of the customer - do a floor-walk at least once a day.

- Keep the merchandising looking full at all times - sparse-looking products do nothing to enhance sales.

- If the space available is greater than the volume of merchandise, keep the presentation tight to the centre - don't try to stretch it out to fill the shelf. Rather like orange juice, the more water you add the more diluted it becomes.

- Keep everything priced - professionally. Little white sticky labels with handwritten pricing has no place in the professional salon or spa, it just looks sloppy and 'bargain basement'.

- Create visual breaks using different shaped products, different coloured packaging or professional merchandising cards.

Tips for effective displays

- Apply the theory that 'less is more' for all displays - it needs to be simple to understand and even simpler to maintain.
- Keep the shape of a pyramid in mind - displays should have a focal point and be balanced either side.
- Use odd numbers for displays - either in groups of three or five.
- For a dramatic or bold display of a very special product, merchandise it on its own - an 'iconic' effect and highly eye-catching.
- Let all retail displays 'tell a story' - customers need to know what they are looking at, what the product's benefits are, where they can buy it and how much it costs.

Great visual merchandising is about common sense and an understanding of your customer.

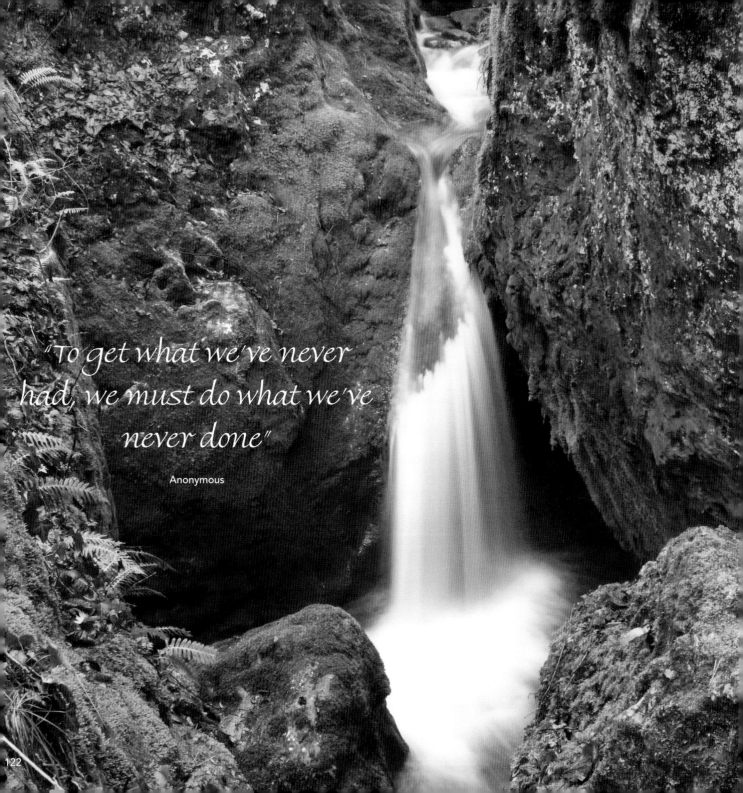

"To get what we've never had, we must do what we've never done"

Anonymous

SOURCES

Arnould-Taylor W (1977) *Principles and Practice of Physical Therapy*. Stanley Thrones Ltd

Begoun P (2002) *The Beauty Bible*. Beginning Press

Carlton Books Limited (2000) *Vogue Beauty*. Carlton Books

Hall J (2002) *The Exercise Bible*. Kyle Cathie Limited

Holford P (1997) *The Optimum Nutrition Bible*. Piatkus Limited

Hora Malhotra R (2005) *Inner Beauty*. Chronicle Books

Lawless J (1995) *The Illustrated Encyclopaedia of Essential Oils*. Element Books

Lawless J (1997) *The Complete Illustrated Guide to Aromatherapy*. Element Books

Marsden K (1993) *Super Skin*. Thorsons

Mehta N & K (2001) *The Art of Indian Face Massage*. Element Books

Norman L (1988) *The Reflexology Handbook*. Piatkus Limited

Reed Gach M (1992) *Acupressure*. Piatkus Limited

The Body Shop International PLC (1994) *The Body Shop Book*. Little, Brown & Company

Wills J (1998) *The Food Bible*. Quadrille Publishing Limited

"Learn as if you were going to live forever, live as though you were going to die tomorrow"

Mahatma Gandhi

SUGGESTED FURTHER READING

Begoun, P (2003) *Don't Go to the Cosmetics Counter Without Me.* Beginning Press

Duncan, Todd (2005) *Sales Motivation.* Simple Truths/Maximum Impact

Duncan, Todd (2005) *The Simple Truths of Selling.* Simple Truths

Element Books (1996) *Alternative Medicine.* Element Books Ltd

Erasmus, U (1986) *Fats that Heal and Fats that Kill.* Alive Books

Glenville, M (1999) *Natural Alternatives to Dieting.* Kyle Cathie Limited

Mortimore, D (1998) *Nutritional Healing.* Element Books

Parker, Sam & Anderson, Mac (2006) 212° *The Extra Degree.* Simple Truths & Walk the Talk

Pitman, V & MacKenzie, K (1997) *Reflexology: A Practical Approach.* Stanley Thrones Ltd

Polunin, M (1997) *Healing Foods.* Dorling Kindersley Ltd

Shapiro, D (1996) *Your Body Speaks Your Mind.* Piatkus Ltd

Vyas, B & Haggard, C (1997) *Beauty Wisdom.* Thorsons

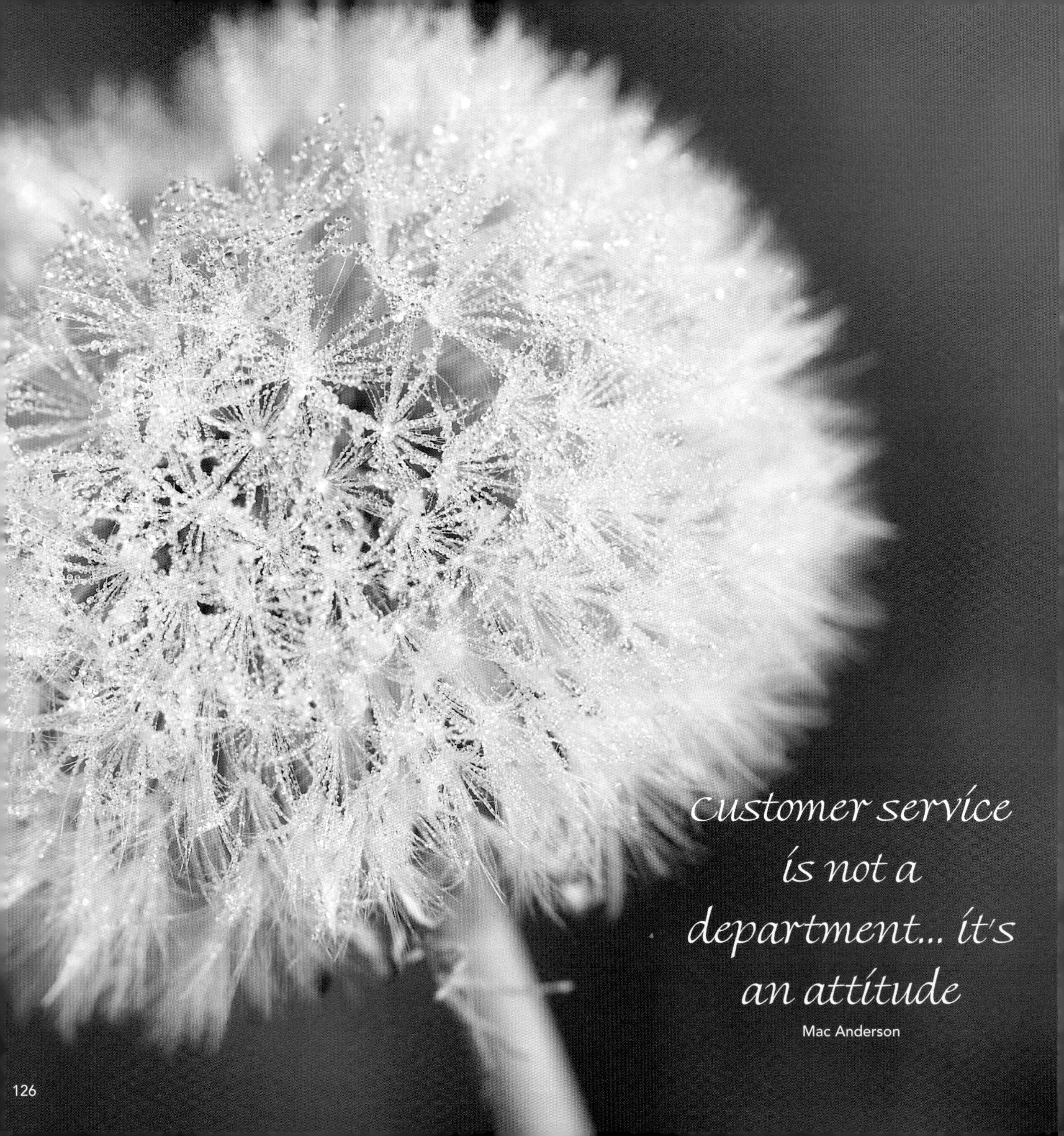

Customer service
is not a
department... it's
an attitude

Mac Anderson

DIRECTORY OF ORGANISATIONS

The Aromatherapy Organisations Council (AOC)
PO Box 19834
London
SE25 6WF

The Association for Therapeutic Healers
79 Brixton Hill
London
SW2 1JF
www.athealers.com

The Association of Chinese Medicine
78 Haverstock Hill
London
NW3 2BE

The Association of Reflexologists
27 Old Gloucester Street
London
WC1N 3XX
www.reflexology.org/aor

The Ayurvedic Company of Great Britain
81 Wimpole Street
London
W1M 7DB

BABTAC Limited
Ambrose House
Meteor Court
Barnett Way
Barnwood
Gloucester
GL4 3GG

The British Complementary Medicine Association
Kensington House
33 Imperial Square
Cheltenham
Gloucestershire
GL50 1QZ
www.bcma.co.uk

The British Massage Therapy Council
78 Meadow Street
Preston
Lancashire
PR1 1TF

Federation of Holistic Therapists (FHT)
18 Shakespeare Business Centre
Hathaway Close
Eastleigh
Hampshire
SO50 4SR

ITEC
2nd floor, Chiswick Gate
598-608 Chiswick High Road
London
W4 5RT

Habia
Oxford House
Sixth Avenue, Sky Business Park
Robin Hood Airport
Doncaster DN9 3GG 0845 2306080

Vocational Training Charitable Trust (VTCT)
www.vtct.org.uk

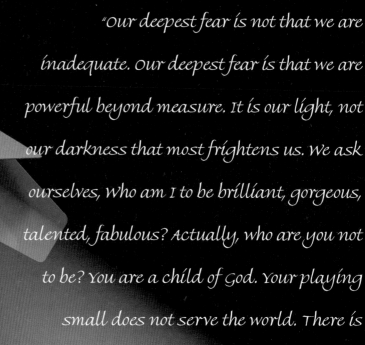

"Our deepest fear is not that we are inadequate. Our deepest fear is that we are powerful beyond measure. It is our light, not our darkness that most frightens us. We ask ourselves, Who am I to be brilliant, gorgeous, talented, fabulous? Actually, who are you not to be? You are a child of God. Your playing small does not serve the world. There is nothing enlightened about shrinking so that other people won't feel insecure around you. We are all meant to shine, as children do. We were born to make manifest the glory of God that is within us. It's not just in some of us; it's in everyone. And as we let our own light shine, we unconsciously give other people permission to do the same. As we are liberated from our own fear, our presence automatically liberates others."

Marianne Williamson from A Return To Love: Reflections on the Principles of A Course in Miracles, published by HarperCollins, 1993. ISBN 9780060923419